WHAT WE KNOW ABOUT CANCER

WHAT WE KNOW ABOUT CANCER

Edited by

R. J. C. HARRIS

London
GEORGE ALLEN & UNWIN LTD
RUSKIN HOUSE   MUSEUM STREET

PRINTED IN GREAT BRITAIN
in 11 on 12 pt. Baskerville
BY CLARKE, DOBLE & BRENDON LTD
PLYMOUTH

The suggestion that a book such as this should be written was first made to the Editor by Jeremy Murray-Brown, who had just produced a most successful television documentary film called *Men Against Cancer*. The idea was timely for another reason. The British Cancer Council, whose object is 'to promote education on the subject of cancer and its prevention, treatment and aftercare', had just come into existence and some of those who had promoted it readily agreed not only to contribute, as experts, to the writing of the book but also to donate all their royalties to help develop the work and influence of the new Council.

We are grateful to Mrs G. M. Dunmore for her help in preparing the material for publication, and we also thank Mr Peter Leek, of Allen and Unwin, for his forbearance with us over the difficulties, for a publisher, inherent in a book with many authors.

CONTENTS

11

GLOSSARY

Ablation

The removal of a part of the body by excision or amputation.

Amino acid

Essential formula is R-CH (NH₂)-COOH where R is a variable chemical group. Combine end to end with each other in hundreds to form proteins. Variations in R leads to the 20 different amino acids found in most proteins.

Ankylosing spondylitis

Inflammation of the vertebrae leading to fixation of the joints.

Antibody

A modified protein in the blood formed by the body in response to, and for the neutralization of, foreign substances known as antigens (q.v.).

Antigen (antigenicity)

Any foreign material (e.g. a viral or bacterial component) which stimulates the formation of antibody (q.v.) when it gains access to an animal's tissues.

Benign tumour

Non-malignant, i.e. unlikely to show invasiveness in adjacent tissues or to metastasize to secondary sites.

Betatron

An accelerator for electrons (q.v.) which produces either a high-energy electron beam, or X-rays.

'Blast' cell

An immature cell, occurring in blood-cell forming tissues, which is a precursor of cells with defined properties.

Carcinogenic

Capable of inducing cancer.

Carcinogenesis

The process by which carcinogens – cancer-inducing materials – convert normal cells to cancer cells.

Choriocarcinoma

A highly malignant cancer arising very rarely from cells which form the junction between the

13

developing embryo and the tissues of the mother's womb.

Curettage

Scraping the interior of an internal cavity, for example the womb, to remove abnormal tissues.

Cyclotron

An accelerator for producing high energy beams of protons (q.v.), *cf.* betatron.

Diathermy

The production of a locally elevated temperature in a tissue produced by a high-frequency electric current. Cauterization.

Ectopic

A tissue, or organ, which is not in its proper place in the body.

Electron

A negatively charged sub-atomic particle. With protons (q.v.) one of the component particles of the atom. About 1/2000th the mass of a hydrogen atom.

Endoplasmic reticulum

A system of fine membrane structures in the cytoplasm of the cell concerned in part with the manufacture of proteins (q.v.) in the cell.

Enzyme

A protein (q.v.), made by the cells, which induces chemical changes in other substances without, itself, being changed. A biological catalyst.

Enzymes, glycolytic

Enzymes in the cell responsible for the breakdown of sugars.

Enzymes, respiratory

Enzymes in the cell responsible for the utilization of oxygen.

Epithelial cells

The cell layer which covers all the free surfaces of tissues in the body, including the glands.

Familial polyposis

Small projecting masses of tissue, which occur in the lower part of the small intestine and colon in members of the same family.

Fistula

An abnormal passage leading to the surface, from an abscess cavity or from a hollow organ, e.g. the bladder.

*Gene
(genetic code)*

The functional unit of heredity. Each gene occupies a specific place in the chromosomes of the cell and reproduces itself exactly at each cell division.

Gonadotrophin

Hormone, from the pituitary gland, which stimulates the genital glands.

Guinea-pig serum

The liquid portion of clotted guinea-pig blood. Will contain antibodies (q.v.) and enzymes (q.v.).

Haemoglobin

The red protein which combines with, and transports, oxygen. Found in the red blood cells.

Herpes virus

One of a group of viruses producing diseases in both animals and man. The lesions are first proliferative and then, usually, necrotic.

Histocompatibility

A state of immunological similarity (or identity) of tissues such that successful transplantation can occur between one individual and another.

Hodgkin's Disease

A disease marked by chronic enlargement of the lymph nodes, first in the neck and then elsewhere, together with enlargement of the spleen.

Homeostasis

Maintenance of the constancy of the internal environment of the cell, tissue or organism.

Homograft

A piece of tissue, or organ, transferred from one member to another member of the same species (but not to an identical twin).

*Hydrocarbon,
polycyclic*

Composed of more than one benzene ring each fused at two points to another, e.g. anthracene, $C_{14}H_{10}$.

Hyperbaric oxygenation	A pressure of oxygen greater than that in normal air.
Hypopharynx	That part of the pharynx which lies below the aperture of the larynx.
Immune reaction	A reaction between antigens (q.v.) and antibodies (q.v.).
Keratin	A sulphur-containing protein (q.v.) found in structures such as hair, nails, horn and the outer surface of the skin.
Latent virus	A virus which is concealed in the cells and tissues but which may be evoked (and thus produce disease) in different ways.
Leukaemia, lymphoblastic	A form of leukaemia (uncontrolled proliferation of the white cell elements of the blood) in which the abnormal cells are those of the blast (q.v.) forms of the lymphocyte (q.v.) series.
Leukaemia, myelogenous	A form of leukaemia characterized by uncontrolled proliferation in the bone-marrow of one of the white blood-cell types.
Linear accelerator	Another machine (like a betatron [q.v.]) for accelerating sub-atomic particles.
Lymph nodes	An organ containing lymphoid tissue, which produces lymphocytes (q.v.).
Lymphoblast	A young, immature cell that becomes a lymphocyte (q.v.).
Lymphocyte	A white blood cell formed in lymphoid tissue throughout the body (e.g. in lymph nodes, spleen, thymus, tonsils).
Lysosome	A cytoplasmic organelle of the cell which contains hydrolysing enzymes (q.v.).
Mammography	Examination of the breast with X-rays.

16

Mastectomy	Amputation of the breast.
Mediastinum	The dividing wall of the chest cavity containing all the structures *except* the lungs.
Metabolism, metabolite	Chemical changes whereby one substance is converted into another in the organism. A metabolite may either be made by the organism or taken from the environment.
Milligram	One-thousandth part of a gramme.
Mitochondria	Microscopic bodies in the cytoplasm of every cell concerned with energy production. Contains many enzyme (q.v.) systems.
Molecular biology	The study of the structure and function of the molecules (such as the nucleic acids and proteins) which are of importance in biology.
Mutation	A change in the character of a gene (q.v.) which is perpetuated in the progeny of the cell in which the change occurred.
Mycoplasma	Disease-producing micro-organisms sometimes called pleuropneumonia-like organisms (PPLO). Have properties related to both bacteria and viruses.
Neuroblastoma	A malignant cancer arising from nerve cells of embryonic type.
Neutrons	Electrically-neutral particle in the atomic nucleus with a mass the same as that of the proton (q.v.).
Nucleated	Containing a cell nucleus, characteristic of all true cells but not, e.g., of mature red blood cells in human blood.
Oesophagus	The portion of the digestive tract between pharynx and stomach.

Otolaryngologist A physician who specializes in the treatment of disorders of the ears and upper respiratory tract.

Pelvimetry Measurement of the diameters of the pelvis.

Pernicious anaemia A chronic progressive disease characterized by reduction of red blood cells in the blood. Administration of vitamin B12 cures this condition if it is uncomplicated.

Placental barrier Small molecules may be exchanged between maternal and embryonic blood in the mammalian placenta, but there is a 'barrier' to the exchange of cells or very large molecules.

Platelet A small cell found in the blood, containing granules but no definite nucleus. Liberates thromboplastin, essential for blood-clotting, when damaged or outside the blood vessels.

Protein Complex chemical compound composed of very large numbers of amino acids (q.v.) joined together. Characteristic of all living systems.

Proton Unit of positive electricity. For hydrogen it is the nucleus of the atom around which a single unit of negative electricity (the electron, q.v.) revolves.

Radioactive isotope Chemically identical atoms of an element which differ in mass number (i.e. their nuclei contain different numbers of neutrons), and which disintegrate spontaneously with the liberation of sub-atomic particles (such as electrons, q.v.) or radiation.

Regeneration Reproduction, or repair, of a lost or injured part.

Resection To cut out a segment of a part, e.g. of the intestine.

18

Retinoblastoma	A malignant cancer arising from the retina of the embryo, usually in very young children.
Roentgen unit	The international unit of X- or gamma-radiation.
Sensitization	A condition in which the response to second and later stimuli is greater than that to the original stimulus (which may indeed have been inapparent).
Steroid hormone	The sex hormone, and hormones of the adrenal cortex closely related chemically to the sterols (q.v.) – e.g. oestrone.
Sterols	Chemical substance built around a four member ring system

– cyclopentanophenanthrene.

Synergistic	Aiding the action of another; for drugs, more than a purely additive effect.
Tissue culture	The growth of cells and tissues in nutrient media outside the body.
Template	A pattern, or guide, that determines the shape of a substance.
Teratogenic	Capable of altering growth processes in an embryo and thus leading to the production of deformities.
Thermography	Production of a regional temperature map (of the breast). Measures radiant heat, and thus blood flow, which can vary in the neighbourhood of tumours.
Toxin	A poisonous substance, usually liberated during the metabolism and growth of bacteria, etc.

19

Ulcerative colitis	A disease of the colon, characterized by ulceration, bleeding, scarring, etc. Unknown origin but thought to dispose to cancer of the colon in some cases.
Wilms' tumour	A malignant cancer of the kidney in young children.

CHAPTER I

CO-OPERATION AND ORGANIZATION IN CANCER RESEARCH AND TREATMENT

GRAHAM BENNETTE

INTRODUCTION

National and international co-operation in cancer research and treatment is not only necessary for the avoidance of expensive duplication of effort by the exchange of data and techniques. It is also *felt* as a compelling need, for there is an intuitive feeling, as well as an intellectual knowledge, that cancer is deeply rooted in fundamental living processes, and these include both the processes which can be studied objectively and, in the human disease, those which are subjectively experienced. Cancer is therefore of concern to every basic scientific discipline in research, and its study pushes forward the frontiers of knowledge. At the personal level the disease is experienced, more or less consciously, as an approach to the frontiers of existence, involving not only the patient but his family and all those who are concerned with the human dilemma of illness.

The latter include, of course, the doctors, the nurses and their colleagues – those who translate the work of the laboratories into human action. They also include the social and public health workers and the educators who are concerned in different ways to translate thought and feeling into action. The different spheres interpenetrate and overlap and one might hope to find a continuity of effective and relevant co-ordination between them all. It should be the ideal situation for creative co-operation because there is such a clear unanimity of purpose and so few of the 'axes to grind' which spoil many attempts to bring co-operation into human affairs.

We must admit, however, that we have not yet achieved a

satisfactory continuity of effective and relevant co-ordination between the different levels of concern. We, of the newly-formed British Cancer Council (and our parent body, the International Union against Cancer), believe that the major difficulty is the ineffectiveness of communication between one branch of cancer study and another, and between the professions and the public.

THE NEED FOR IMPROVED COMMUNICATION

In the United Kingdom there are dozens of organizations, institutions, committees and charities directly concerned with all aspects of cancer, not only laboratory research establishments and research departments in hospitals, but also societies, trusts and other foundations which concentrate on the problems of the care of patients and their families. There are also many organizations devoted to cancer education and prevention. All these bodies are independent and are financed, for the most part, by voluntary contributions.

We are probably fortunate to have such a degree of diversity and thus to avoid the difficulties inherent in a system which is unified in its administrative, financial and policy structure. The main advantage is that cancer studies at every level depend upon an exploratory approach as well as a systematic one, and the exploration and testing of new ideas and techniques demands as much freedom as possible, freedom from the sort of centralized direction that can so easily inhibit inventiveness.

It is often argued, of course, that a multiplicity of independent working units is uneconomical. In the straightforward programmes of work which expand in the wake of new concepts — filling in the details and working out the applications by systematic development, this may be so. Explorers are not required to be 'efficient' and 'economical', but those who follow them to survey and develop the new territory must collaborate efficiently, by integrating their work and avoiding duplication of effort. At the level of exploration we cannot afford to be too economical: at the other level of development and exploitation, we cannot afford not to be. We need to find a system of communication and organization in which both kinds of opportunity can be pursued fully, and this is what the new British Cancer Council aims to do.

The problem of diversity is, of course, the problem of communication, and this is especially difficult in cancer studies because they are so complex. The specialists in the many different branches speak different 'technical languages' – often so different that it takes too long for busy scientists, doctors and social workers to undertake the task of 'translation'. The enormous rate at which knowledge is accumulating adds to the difficulty, so that the specialist finds it increasingly difficult to keep up with advances in his own area of work. Inevitably, then, specialization tends to increase. There is an urgent need to find ways to make a broader view accessible to people, to compensate for this situation in which the individual workers have to concentrate on smaller and smaller parts of the whole subject, making it impossible for them to exploit the maximum potential of their special fields of study.

PERSONAL FACTORS IN COMMUNICATION AND CO-OPERATION

What do we mean when we refer to 'the cancer problem'? Any illness may be regarded, from the personal point of view, primarily as a situation of crisis. It is a crisis of suffering or at least of difficulty. Cancer is more than a complicated collection of biological, medical and social problems calling for solutions, it is also a human situation that calls for help. The people who are ill obviously need help – but so do those who are helping the ones who are ill.

There are a great many definable problems of cancer that can certainly be solved by science and medicine : many have been solved by painstaking, specialized work, and many more will be solved in the future. But there are difficulties in the whole situation of illness which cannot be solved simply by increasing the number of specialized scientific studies. These are aspects of the total situation of the people who are involved in the illness, both the patients and the helpers. It has to do with the personal and essentially human experience and dilemma of illness.

It is a platitude to say that we must take care not to lose sight of the individual in our concern to help the patient to cope with his crisis by concentrating only on the technical and tangible means at our disposal. Perhaps it is less of a platitude to say that we must not lose sight of the individual in our efforts, at the level of organization, to help the scientists, doctors and social workers to cope with their dilemmas by concentrating only on the technical expertise of the system of organization.

For the patient in the hospital bed, cancer is not just a complex set of scientific, medical and social problems. He will feel that *he has* been overlooked if he is approached mainly as a problem to be solved. For the busy scientist and doctor, who is held down by the sheets and sheets of scientific papers, books, reviews and abstracts, quite as securely as by any hospital counterpane, the same feeling can be true. Cancer organization can become just one more burden, another load of paper threatening sanity, if it is mediated by impersonal, faceless committees, or ponderous administrative machines.

Administrative or organizational structure is an anatomy which is of no interest to anyone (except the administrative anatomist) unless it is *alive*. What gives it life and the capacity to translate thought and feeling into action? Can the 'problems' of organizational design be 'solved' merely by slipping in another Joint Standing Committee? It may become very ingeniously articulated by such devices, and it may stand – albeit rather unsteadily – but it will not necessarily be alive and well and living in Geneva. This is where the International Union against Cancer has its headquarters. It is the feeling of participation that counts, in which the people who take part also give a part.

This feeling exists in the International Union more strongly than ever before, and it is the same feeling that has brought the British Cancer Council into being. Why else should so many leading people – and very busy people, from dozens of organizations – so enthusiastically grasp at the chance to co-operate more closely? I am sure that there is here a shared conviction that it is possible, by improved translation and communication, to bring knowledge into closer contact with experience, leading to a greater understanding and more effective action.

THE TRANSLATION AND DIRECTION OF INFORMATION

The translation of information sounds complicated but straightforward enough, and at the practical level of information exchange, so it is. But there is also a vital aspect here in which the same intangible factors of feeling and intuition can play a major part. It is the question of *how* the information is collected and to *whom* it is distributed.

Nowadays no one can know very much about anything and we turn hopefully, but with some misgivings, towards the computers with their rapid information retrieval. The misgivings arise because we know that computers cannot give simple answers to complicated questions—and not always to simple ones. Information is accumulating so fast and the confidence that can be placed in some of it is so questionable that we will be scarcely any better off in a few years time when the computerized libraries will provide us with a hundred or so references in response to a question about cancer, where it is difficult or impossible to frame an enquiry in a highly-specific way.

There is another possibility—the old-fashioned one of personal communication. What no computer can do is to drop someone a line or ring him up and ask nicely. A small group of trained individuals in touch with a large and reliable panel of those who really know all that is relevant in every branch of the subject can exchange information more rapidly than any computer. We shall certainly need the computers, but we shall also need a new breed of retriever—information officers who will take on some of the burden of selecting, reviewing and translating from one specialized language to another. They will be the antithesis of the specialists in that they will need to know a little about a great deal, with an awareness of the very different information needs of those working on different aspects of the disease. They will have to judge whom to ask and where to direct the information.

The *direction* of the information flow raises another important question. Because we are all facing the same way in trying to help the patient, we are inclined to accept the idea of a sort of hierarchy in which the scientist tells the doctor about his results, and the doctor then applies these to the care of his patient—with a good many intermediate steps on the way, of course. Most scientists and doctors would agree that this process of communication also needs to operate in the other direction. If the greater specialist were to have more access to the experience of the lesser, it would doubtless be found that there is still a great deal that the doctors can learn from their patients and the scientists can learn from the doctors.

So far as the latter case is concerned, scientists have been concentrating for decades on the early stages of *primary* cancer and particularly on the mechanisms of its induction and natural origin. This is obviously a sensible fundamental approach, but there has been a general lack of emphasis in experimental research on the processes of the *secondary* spread of the disease. Scientists must give more acknowledgement to the fact, so clear to doctors, that early primary cancer never killed anyone.

One of the most direct ways in which patients can collaborate with doctors is in the field of rehabilitation, by helping them to find ways of improving the methods to overcome the handicaps that may result from treatment. An example of this is a group which was founded in the United States that is doing very valuable work in helping women who have to face the problems of breast removal as a result of a cancer. Carefully selected volunteers who have recovered from the same operation collaborate with the hospital staff in giving practical feminine help and support to those facing the same difficulties. From their personal experience they can give advice on some of the small but very important problems. They come to the patient's bedside, neatly, fashionably and conspicuously dressed in jersey dresses. With more time to spend than the doctors and nurses could afford, they can put new heart into people who could so easily surrender in the struggle to keep up appearances and make the necessary efforts to live more fully. They give advice on how to get improved artificial breast forms, how to alter clothes and still keep one step ahead of fashion, and how to do the exercises that will, for example, make it easier for the convalescent patient to do her hair.

There has proved to be no shortage of sensible and sensitive women for this task – women who have gained the confidence of the doctors and who can uniquely gain the confidence of the patients. Many others engaged in different fields of cancer rehabilitation contribute in similar ways, mobilizing the will to live and helping patients to return to normal life.

THE INTERNATIONAL UNION AGAINST CANCER

Before describing what is being done and what we aim to do in a practical way in the British Cancer Council, we should look at the developments which have led to the present activities of the

International Union against Cancer – the UICC for short (from the initial letters of its title in French).

The plan to form an International Union against Cancer developed over several years in the 1920s and earlier, but it was not until the First International Cancer Congress in Madrid in 1933 that the Union was officially established. Since then there have been eight International Congresses, at each of which there has been a steadily improving participation among the representatives of cancer studies in all its aspects from an increasing number of nations. The Seventh International Cancer Congress was held at the Festival Hall in London in 1958, and many believe that this occasion was a turning point in the development of international co-operation. So great was the expansion of interest and activity after this Congress – and in no small measure because of it – that it became necessary for the Union to formulate a much wider Constitution, and this occurred at the last Cancer Congress, in Tokyo in 1966.

The Union now has seventy member countries and it has been very disappointing that the contribution made by the United Kingdom has declined rather than increased in recent years. It is all the more disappointing when one considers the impetus that was given by the organizers in this country at the time of the Seventh Congress. By 1967 the subscription from Britain to the UICC had fallen to a derisory figure – the most that could be raised by our national cancer research society, the British Association for Cancer Research, which hurriedly filled the breach when the former British National Committee on Cancer was disbanded soon after the Tokyo Congress.

It was this inadequacy in our national contribution to the UICC that provided one major reason for bringing the new British Cancer Council into being, and the Council is now committed to fulfil the national responsibility to give both ideas, work and funds to the international efforts of the UICC. It has been said that we in Britain – on a population basis – have a greater potential of advanced ideas and techniques in cancer studies than any other country in the world. We have a lot to give in these ways, but, being one of the ten richest nations on earth, we must surely find the means to back up the ideas with an adequate contribution of money as well.

Apart from any questions of moral obligation or prestige, it is

27

quite simply the soundest investment that can be made to guarantee that advances are rapid. Recent developments carry that guarantee. There are always a few people, of course, entrenched in an attitude of isolated specialization and general cynicism, who will argue that international effort is hopeless and clumsy. They will say that it is nothing more than a glorious way for non-productive, or even counter-productive, old men to have innumerable trips to romantic places in order to mumble banalities in some unrealistic, polyglot committee – and thereafter to enjoy whatever delights may be offered by the foreign city in question. It could be like this, but no one with any contemporary grasp of the significance of current international research collaboration could take such a point of view seriously.

Perhaps the most exciting example of such international collaboration at the present time was started in Uganda, where Mr Denis Burkitt described cases of a hitherto unrecognized form of childhood cancer. It will probably never be justified to talk about a 'breakthrough' in cancer in the way suggested by some over-enthusiastic reporters, but if ever there were an international communications breakthrough, I think it is Burkitt's tumour that must be seen as the spearhead. From East Africa to London, to Stockholm and Paris, to New York and New Guinea, to Bristol and Philadelphia, to Australia and Minneapolis, and back again to Africa, the dialogues are carried on between every kind of specialist – physicians, radiotherapists, surgeons, pathologists, chemotherapists, virus experts, immunologists, epidemiologists and statisticians. This is an extraordinary phenomenon of communication and the results which are emerging are not only relevant to a cancer in African children – although some of these have come off miraculously well, too. The results have the most far-reaching and fundamental significance to a better grasp of the meaning of the cancer process as a whole, offering clues to a greater knowledge of a number of other, quite unexpected problems, and probably giving important insights into the basic mechanisms of immunity as well. These are the sort of dividends that international co-operation can guarantee.

Of the seventy countries represented in the UICC there are few with so much to give as Britain. In the history of cancer research the British contribution has been outstanding and today the important new direction of research into Burkitt's tumour was pioneered by British cancer workers. But the rate at which these problems can be pursued now depends on international effort, to which British research workers continue to make contributions of decisive significance. Now that the pursuit of these exciting ideas is branching out in a way that involves many people in other countries, it is very important that these nations should support their countrymen by giving money to the Union, the organization that is doing so much to promote and co-ordinate the work. One of the functions of the new British Cancer Council will be the raising of money to pay a proper British share to the Union. The proceeds of this book will be devoted to this and to the work of the Council at a national level, through the generosity and commitment of the Editor and the others who have contributed.

The Union currently works through Commissions which cover the whole field of cancer, and it is evidence that our contribution of ideas is highly valued that two of these Commissions currently have British Chairmen, and others from this country take part in the various study groups. There is not enough space here to describe the work of all the Commissions and study groups, but the Commission on Fellowships should be given special mention because it answers so concretely the question 'What can the Union do for us?'. During the period 1961 to 1967, workers in this country were either given grants by the Union to travel abroad and increase their knowledge and experience, or were given assistance in their home laboratories from overseas workers to the total value of £135,000. It is a sad commentary on the level of our national contribution to have to say that this is about six times more than Britain gave to the UICC during this period.

The Secretary-General of the UICC has recently answered the question 'What can the Union do for its members?' in the following terms. Because of its very extensive membership and contacts, the Union can offer expert advice in the fields of organization, public education, professional education, the organization of cancer detection and treatment programmes and the co-ordination of many research activities. It also offers the research fellowships already mentioned, and provides the means of communication between its member organizations by arranging congresses, conferences and symposia. It publishes and distributes a leading scientific journal, the *International Journal*

29

of Cancer, and sends out monographs, technical reports and regular bulletins of international information.

THE BRITISH CANCER COUNCIL

The British Cancer Council has been broadly modelled on the basic structure of the International Union, and functions through an Executive Committee consisting of representatives of leading people in this country in clinical research, experimental research, hospital diagnosis and treatment, relief and rehabilitation, terminal care, prevention and detection, and education. An independent Finance Committee will raise the necessary funds by private subscription to meet our international obligations and to find the resources to staff and equip a central office. The Council will not be a fund-raising body in order to finance research projects and no public appeals will be made. These aspects of cancer work are already admirably undertaken by several of the independent organizations that are represented on the Council.

The Council was inaugurated on June 12, 1968 under the presidency of Professor Sir John Bruce, and its Constitution was adopted in November, 1968. At present there are thirty-eight organizations participating and these are represented by a total of sixty-six members or observers. Observers have been appointed by the Ministry of Health, the Scottish Home and Health Department, the Ministry of Health and Social Services of Northern Ireland, the Medical Research Council, the Health Education Council and the Biological Council. Several other organizations have been invited to join, and there is every reason to anticipate that the Council will soon be able to bring together every cancer organization in Britain and will become the centre for information and advice for everyone.

The central office is intended to provide a national information service and will maintain contacts within the country at every level of cancer work. These will be drawn together and brought into closer touch with the International Union, and information from the Union will be distributed through the Council to its member organizations.

The Council is also arranging meetings and study groups. Three such groups have been established so far: one on advanced

30

cancer care, another in which new ideas on cancer rehabilitation will be developed, and a third on information processing in the cancer field. Advisory reports will be issued when the work has advanced sufficiently. These discussions will include many members who are not directly associated with the Council, and the subjects will be chosen in order to provide the maximum opportunity for people in different areas of work to co-operate. Other groups are envisaged: for example to study ways of improving communications; to investigate the problems of 'resistance' to cancer education that so seriously limit the effectiveness of the preventive measures that can be taken for certain forms of cancer; and yet another will explore new experimental possibilities for studying the processes of the secondary spread of the disease.

The Council will keep in touch with representatives of the press, radio and television and will try to provide authoritative answers or opinions to anyone looking for information who is seriously interested in making a contribution in any field of the work. We believe that this is especially important if we are to check some of the myths that confuse people and give rise to false fears and false hopes. This book is our first attempt to talk about the complexities of the whole subject in a language that demands a minimum of special training on the part of the reader. Already we have published the proceedings of the first Symposia organized by the Council. This booklet deals with some of the less technical aspects of cancer, also translated in a way that will be easily intelligible to everyone.

Sir David Smithers referred to the urgent need to improve communication by improving intelligibility, in his inaugural address to the Council. He went on to say, 'It may be that one of the greatest weaknesses in our cancer enterprise stems from the difficulty in exchanging information and experience. Vital knowledge has been available in many fields for many years before its significance has sparked a response in the proper quarter. The "Eureka Principle" needs to be remembered as never before in an age of such intensive specialization. A typewriter and a telephone may not seem as impressive as an electron microscope or a linear accelerator, but they are nonetheless indispensable if the electron microscopists are to talk to radiotherapists and clinicians to microbiologists. These simple and inexpensive instruments of communication in the proper hands can help to create the

31

conditions in which new ideas can arise and be tested, and from which fresh opportunities for practical help for ordinary people can emerge.'

'We hope to find through this Council more effective ways of bringing the many specialists from the laboratory and bedside at the scientific, practical and personal levels to open up new approaches to the many human problems created by cancer. Our wide membership will make sure that all aspects of specialized work and all ventures of community care will be joined in our discussions. I believe that we have here one of the most promising –and, in these difficult times, one of the most economical– prospects of advance in our subject. Not just our subject as cancer workers, but our subject as part of the community. We need not only greater knowledge but also a greater understanding of these problems that all too frequently come near to our homes. The Cancer Council should succeed in advancing general under-standing–so reducing fear–and at the same time advance particular understanding so that knowledge gained may be more quickly and effectively applied to the needs of patients.'

The concern of the Council with these personal and essentially human aspects of the situation of crisis is shown in the title of its first Symposium, 'People and Cancer', in which the contributions were devoted to the intangible questions as well as the practical ones–to the attitudes towards the disease, to the personal relation-ship between the doctor or nurse and the patient, and to the patients' special needs, physical, psychological and spiritual. All of these approaches are included in the title of the closing lecture, 'The Care of the Individual'.

I would like to sum up these remarks on co-operation and organization by telling the Hasidic story of the Rabbi who was having a conversation with the Lord about Heaven and Hell. 'I will show you Hell,' said the Lord and led the Rabbi into a room in the middle of which was a very big round table. The people sitting at it were famished and desperate. In the middle of the table there was a large pot of stew, enough and more for everyone. The smell of the stew was delicious and made the Rabbi's mouth water. The people round the table were holding spoons with very long handles. Each one found that it was just possible to reach the pot to take a spoonful of the stew, but because the handle of his spoon was longer than a man's arm, he could not get the food back into his mouth. The Rabbi saw that their suffering was terrible. 'Now I will show you Heaven,' said the Lord, and they went into another room exactly the same as the first. There was the same big round table and the same pot of stew. The people, as before, were equipped with the same long-handled spoons – but here they were well nourished and plump, laughing and talking. At first the Rabbi could not understand. 'It is simple, but it requires a certain skill,' said the Lord. 'You see, they have learned to feed each other.'

It will be our business in the Council to find ways to feed each other with knowledge, and as far as we can, with understanding and concern. But to say that we will try to feed each other does not mean ourselves alone, the ones directly involved in the committees and study groups, but everyone who wants to see the words 'community care' really mean something.

When the Council was first proposed, several people understandably reacted by saying, 'What! *another* cancer organization? Haven't we got enough already?' I hope that this introductory chapter has shown that the Council will not be just one more cancer organization. It is an attempt to draw together the existing ones – the 'organs' of cancer work – into a corporate whole, into an *organism*. We may then hope to transmit something of its vitality to the people who are ill.

CHAPTER II

THE NATURE OF CANCER

L. G. LAJTHA

Cancer, or more precisely malignant growth, is defined as a disorder in which some cell type in the organism begins to grow in an apparently unchecked fashion. During this proliferation the cell type – irrespective of the tissue of its origin – tends to lose or change some of its normal biochemical characteristics. In addition, as a result of such changes, cancer cells do not form simple well-isolated tumours, but tend to infiltrate neighbouring tissue, and also tend to spread into distant areas in the body, thus forming 'secondary deposits' or metastases.

It has been realized for some time by doctors and scientists that cancer is not *a* disease. There are many different forms of malignant growth, caused by different agents, having different biochemical properties and requiring different treatments. The definition of cancer given above is therefore a very general one : it describes the common properties of cancerous growths, but it does not help in understanding why or how such disorders can come about, or how they should be dealt with once they have arisen.

In the following pages we shall discuss these basic properties of cancer : growth which is not properly checked and changes in normal cellular biochemical functions, including the property of spreading.

I GROWTH

Growth simply means enlargement. When it comes to talking about cells it is not a very precise term because it could mean enlargement of a cell (or cell type) or increase in number of a cell type. Although cancer cells can be frequently larger than normal cells, malignant growth means increase in number rather than size. The better term for this is proliferation.

34

Cellular proliferation is a normal, indeed essential, property of any organism. It starts in the fertilized egg, proceeds at a fabulous rate during the early stages of embryonic growth, then it begins to slow down with the maturity and development of the organism. By adult life there will be some organs with practically no proliferative capacity (for example the brain), others will maintain a fairly high production of new cells through-out life (for example the bone marrow or the epithelial lining of the gut). There will be also organs or tissues which will proliferate only slowly and only according to demand for new cells (for example, skin which can increase its proliferation considerably during wound healing).

To understand cellular growth we have to understand some of the basic structures in the cell.

(a) The basic anatomy of the cell

All cells consist of two basic structures: the nucleus and the cytoplasm. The nucleus is usually a round body, of about 7–15 microns (0·007–0·015 cm.) in diameter. It is particularly rich in proteins and in two very important substances, nucleic acids: RNA (ribonucleic acid) and DNA (deoxyribonucleic acid). The cytoplasm surrounds the nucleus, it also contains proteins and nucleic acids, but most of its nucleic acids are of the RNA type; only small traces of DNA are present in the cytoplasm. It also contains a number of different small structures, so-called cellular organelles, such as mitochondria, lysosomes, endoplasmic reti-culum, etc., organelles for the specific biochemical functions of the cell. Most of the enzymes, the tools with which the cell can perform chemical reactions, are also usually located in the cyto-plasm surrounding the nucleus.

It is known now, that the key to the identity of the cell is in the nucleus: the substance called nuclear DNA. Although the amount of DNA in a mammalian cell is only about 10^{-8} mg. (= 0·00000000001 gramme), it consists of a very thin double helix (like a twisted ladder) which if it could be stretched out would be about 3 feet long.

The chemical composition of this helix is reasonably simple, it has four basic constituents, the purines, adenine and guanine, and the pyrimidines, cytosine and thymine. These are the four bases, each coupled with a sugar, deoxyribose. The sugar-base

35

complex is called a nucleoside. A phosphate bond connects two sugar molecules (the base-sugar-phosphate complex is called a nucleotide) and two of the bases also bind to each other : adenine with thymine and guanine with cytosine. The structure then looks something like this :

$$
\begin{array}{cc}
| & | \\
\text{deoxyribose} - \text{adenine} = \text{thymine} - \text{deoxyribose} \\
| & | \\
\text{phosphate} & \text{phosphate} \\
| & \\
\text{deoxyribose} - \text{guanine} = \text{cytosine} - \text{deoxyribose} \\
| & | \\
\text{phosphate} & \text{phosphate} \\
| & |
\end{array}
$$

This structure forms a 'twisted ladder' and the rungs of this ladder are the base pairs, adenine–thymine or thymine–adenine, or guanine–cytosine or cytosine–guanine. These base pairs are denoted by the letters A–T, T–A, G–C and C–G.

The combination of sequences of A–T, T–A, G–C and C–G base pairs in the long DNA double helix is the 'genetic code'. It is this sequence which has all the basic determining information in it for the cell (Figure 1). In the different cells various parts of the 'code' may be temporarily (or permanently) repressed, i.e. non-functional. It is the basic code which determines whether a cell is a human cell, a mouse cell or a plant cell, and it is the specific repression pattern in a human cell which determines whether it is a liver, skin or brain cell.

The DNA of a human cell is not a continuous long fibre, it is 'packaged' into forty-six structures called chromosomes. Since each chromosome thus contains some 2–3 cm. length of DNA and considerable amounts of RNA and protein as well, and since

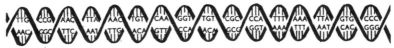

DNA DOUBLE HELIX

FIGURE 1

Scheme of the DNA double helix. The genetic 'code' is the series of bases on one of the strands, three bases being a three-letter 'word' coding for an amino acid, e.g. TTG – GGC – AAC – AAT, etc.

36

forty-six chromosomes are packed into a nucleus of some 7–15 microns in diameter, it can be imagined that some very complex coiling, supercoiling, folding and superfolding of the DNA fibres is necessary to achieve such 'packing'.

(b) Cell division

Cellular proliferation is achieved by cell division. This means that a cell divides into two : the result is two 'daughter' cells which are identical with each other, and identical with the mother cell which had divided. The only way the daughter cells can be identical is by having the same amount and type of DNA in both. Therefore, before a cell can divide in a normal way, the amount of DNA in it has to be duplicated. In a cell which is preparing for cell division the DNA double helices begin to 'open up' and each of the two strands of the helix will act as a template on which new DNA is laid down. In this respect each chromosome behaves as if it would consist of a double helix, and when the cell divides into two, each of the daughter cells will have exactly 50 per cent 'old' and 50 per cent 'new' DNA in them. Indeed in every cell, 50 per cent of the DNA is the result of new DNA synthesis during the last cell cycle (cell cycle is the time between two cell divisions). However, this 'semi-conservative' duplication of the DNA means that DNA is, at least theoretically, imperishable as long as cell divisions go on, and there will be cells with some DNA in them which may have been synthesized (laid down) hundreds of cell cycles before. Furthermore, since DNA is handed down from generation to generation during fertilization of the egg cell by the sperm, some DNA molecules may be present in all of us which are many generations old.

Of course, cell division is a very complex chain reaction or series of complex biochemical processes. First, the cell has to manufacture enzymes – specific chemical tools – with which it can start opening the DNA chain; enzymes with which it can make the building blocks of the new DNA, enzymes with which it can assemble the new DNA. To illustrate the speed of the processes involved and the efficiency required, about 250,000 base pairs (of the A–T or G–C type) have to be assembled *per second* in a mammalian cell during its period of DNA duplication.

Apart from the synthesis of DNA, the cell has to make sufficient extra RNA and protein (and of course again enzymes

37

for their manufacture) to provide material for two cells, and finally it has to manufacture enzymes to build up a last complex process which is called mitosis, the actual process during which the cell divides into two. During this process the chromosomes condense so that they become visible under a good microscope, then they line up in the middle of the cell, and then fine fibres begin to pull them apart towards the two poles of the cell (which begins to elongate at that time). This separation of the chromosomes is done in a way which ensures that both the separated sets of chromosomes are identical, i.e. contain 50 per cent new and 50 per cent old DNA of exactly identical composition. As a last step the cytoplasm is 'pinched in' at the middle and two separate but identical cells take the place of the original one (Figure 2).

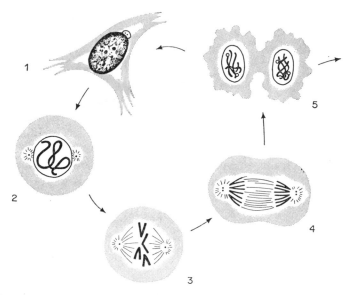

FIGURE 2
Cell division
1. Resting cell.
2. Prophase, the chromosomes become visible.
3. Metaphase, the chromosomes condense and line up in the middle of the cell.
4. Anaphase, the chromosomes separate from each other.
5. Telophase, the chromosomes reconstitute new nuclei and the cell divides into two cells.

(c) Cell populations

Starting from one cell, the fertilized egg, a whole series of different cell populations arise during embryonic development. This is the result of a combination of proliferation and differentiation. Differentiation may be defined as a qualitative change in the biochemical properties of a cell. Such changes are regulated by the DNA : various parts of the 'code' being repressed or de-repressed may disallow or allow the expression of the 'message' in that part of the code. The initiation of such repressions or de-repressions are obviously mediated by certain 'signals' between the cells. For example : the fertilized egg starts proliferation, and after a number of cell divisions – from one cell to two, to four, to eight, to sixteen, etc. – a critical number of cells will exist in this population. At that stage, some of the cells will suffer an event of de-repression, whereby they will acquire some new biochemical properties. They will nevertheless go on proliferating thus creating a second cell population co-existing with the first. In fact the whole of embryonic development is the development of series of new cell populations. These cell populations constitute the various organs and tissues of the organism.

In the adult organism, therefore, a very large number of different cell populations exist. These can be classified on anatomical or biochemical grounds, i.e. liver cells, skin epithelium cells, connective tissue cells, salivary gland cells, insulin-producing pancreatic cells, etc. In the blood-forming organ, the bone marrow, there are again several cell populations : red cell precursors, white cell precursors, precursors of antibody-forming cells, etc.

Looking at these from the point of view of their growth potential one can divide cell populations into certain subclasses, irrespective of their specific anatomical situation or biochemical function. Some of the most important population types are as follows :

1. Closed dividing population. The term 'closed' means that no cells enter the population from elsewhere, nor are cells leaving the population. Leaving means not so much moving from one anatomical location to another, it means loss of cells either because of cell death or physical removal from the body, or loss due to differentiation, i.e. by the cells changing to another type

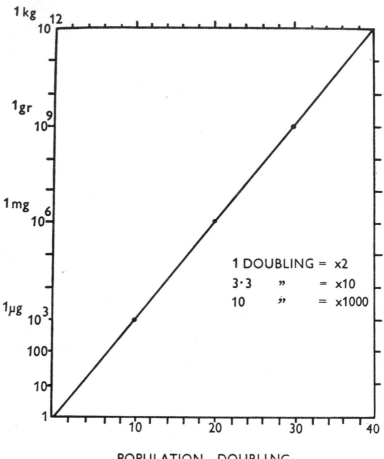

POPULATION DOUBLING

FIGURE 3

Exponential, or logarithmic, growth of a cell population with average size cells in it. One million cells in this case may weight about 1 mg. Large liver cells may weigh twice as much, small lymphocytes half as much.

of cell. Since in the closed dividing population there is no cell removal, but there is continuing cell division, such populations increase their size, usually in an exponential (or logarithmic fashion).

The cells arising from the first few post-fertilization divisions represent such a population, also some tumours in the early stages of their growth may represent such a population. Otherwise such populations do not exist in the body. However, cells grown in tissue cultures are good examples of closed dividing populations.

It might be appropriate to discuss here some facts about exponential growth. It means that at each cell division the whole population doubles: 1, 2, 4, 8, 16, 32, 64, 128, and so on. In other words, after one 'doubling' there are 2 cells, after six doublings 64 cells, after ten doublings about 1,000 cells, as illustrated in Figure 3. It is worthwhile to remember, that twenty doublings give 1,000,000 cells which is barely 1 mg. weight, thirty doublings give 1,000,000,000 cells which may weigh 1 gramme, while forty doublings would reach 1,000,000,000,000 cells weighing almost 1 kg. To give a visual example, if we could set up a single cell which can divide at every twelve hours, and we could keep observing it it would take twenty doublings, i.e. ten days, before one could see a small speck with the naked eye; within the next five days it would grow to the size of a small grape, and a further five days would see the development of a lump the size of a melon. The mistaken illusion would be that for fifteen days there was a slow growth (to the size of a small grape) but it has accelerated in the last five days (to the size of a melon). In fact, the growth rate was the same all the time: one population doubling every twelve hours.

2. Dividing transit population. Such cell populations are the results of differentiation. The essential feature of such populations is that the cells do not remain the same throughout successive cell divisions. This is best illustrated with the nucleated red cell precursor series, the cells destined to produce the mature red cells. At an early stage a process of differentiation (probably gene de-repression resulting in some biochemical change) started in these cells and proceeds at a reasonably fast rate. In the case of the red cell precursors the process is the synthesis of haemoglobin. The rate at which haemoglobin is synthesized is faster than could be diluted or maintained by the successive cell divisions: for example, after the first cell cycle the concentration of haemoglobin may be 14 'units' per cell. After cell division the two identical daughter cells will have 7 units each. However, further synthesis during the next cell cycle may treble this concentration to 21 units per cell – a concentration reached

41

just before the next cell division. After that division there will
be two identical daughter cells with 10·5 units of haemoglobin
in each. During each cell cycle the concentration of haemoglobin
will increase in the cell until it has reached such a high concentration that the cell cannot divide any more. At that stage the cell
will lose its nucleus and turn into an ordinary red cell which will
circulate in the blood for about 110 days.

Another example of such a population is the keratinizing
epithelium of the skin. Again a compound, in this case keratin,
is being built in the cells faster than it can be diluted by the
normal cell divisions. Since the fully keratinized skin cells are
continuously lost from the surface of the skin, a steady supply

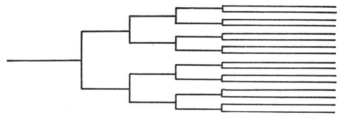

FIGURE 4

Scheme of a dividing transit cell population. It will remain a transit
population only if the concentration of some cell component is increasing
or decreasing. Both these processes will lead to eventual elimination of the
cell. If, however, there is no change in any cell component, this population
would grow exponentially, forming a tumour.

Concentration of 'X' Constant = Exponential Growth
Decreasing = Dedifferentiation
Increasing = Differentiation, Maturation

of differentiating cells is at any time in the 'pipeline' of cell
production.

It is important to realize one aspect of these dividing transit
populations. They come from somewhere, from a special stem
population (to be discussed later) and they go somewhere, either
into the blood or on to the surface of the skin. They will die or
be lost in either case. Consequently, the differentiation results in
a 'suicide pathway' for these cells. Either some compound is
increasing in them (as shown in Figure 4) in which case they will
kill themselves by reaching a critical concentration, or some compound is decreasing in them, in which case they may kill them-

selves by reaching a minimal critical concentration (as probably happens with some white blood cells). This 'suicide' pathway of differentiation (or de-differentiation) is an essential feature of the transit population. If such differentiation would not result in an increase or decrease of a compound in these cells, a compound whose concentration – high or low – would eventually limit the life of the cells, then we would be dealing with an exponentially growing, increasing cell population : a tumour. In other words, the fact that dividing transit populations – like many of our bone-marrow cells – do not turn into tumours, in spite of their high division rate, is due to the suicide pathway of differentiation which maintains them as steady state populations.

3. Stem type populations. By adult life there will be many cell populations – such as liver cells, various glandular cells which do not divide at a fast rate, because there is no loss of cells from the population to any significant extent. Since there is no such thing as a perfect organism, occasional biochemical accidents do happen, and the odd cell does die in any cell population. Since this cell death is likely to be a slow but continuing phenomenon, these slowly dividing cell populations will consist of two functional

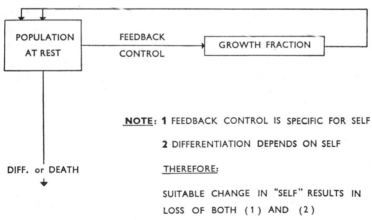

FIGURE 5

Scheme of a stem type of cell population. Part of the population is at rest, from this, occasional cell removal – differentiation or cell death – takes place. To compensate for this, a fraction of the population is proliferating. The control of the size of the cell population and of the differentiation depends on the biochemical identity of the cell. If this changes, both controls may be lost and uncontrolled growth may ensue.

43

states: one at rest, and the other in the process of growth (Figure 5).

It is very important to realize that normal liver, for example, can grow at a fast rate, if and when there is such a demand (e.g. after surgical removal of a large part of the liver). Such increased growth, usually following a demand for regeneration, is regulated by some kind of 'feedback control' of the population size. In other words, there is some mechanism which recognizes whether the size of the cell population is too low or just right. In the first instance, an increasing proportion of cells will be allowed to go into cell division, until such time that the population size is back to normal, when cell division drops to the normal, very low levels.

These populations are called 'stem type' because they usually maintain a line (stem line) of cells. It is the liver cells which maintain their own line of liver cells, or breast gland epithelium maintaining its own line of gland cells. In the bone marrow there is also a stem cell line, a line which maintains itself in spite of differentiation removing some cells from it to create the bone-marrow dividing transit populations described earlier.

It has been said that these cell populations have a specific 'size controlling' mechanism. Such a size control must depend on the recognition of the cell type concerned. If a recognition works on a liver cell population, it will not be able to 'note' differences in a bone-marrow stem cell population. Similarly, the bone-marrow stem cell population size control will not notice whether the liver cells are in normal or subnormal numbers. Therefore, if a bone-marrow stem cell suffers some change, a change which results in changing the essential identity of that cell, then the specific population size control mechanism will not work on such a cell. It may not even respond to stimuli of differentiation, since those also depend on the specific 'self' of a cell population (e.g. a factor called erythropoietin, can induce differentiation in a specific cell population sensitive to it, but not in any other cell population).

The loss or change of the essential 'self' of such stem cell populations results in growth which is not controlled by the specific feedback control mechanism, and also probably in loss of capacity to differentiate into normal useful cells, or, in other words, a tumour.

4. Tumour cell populations. To compare tumour growth with normal tissue growth, the only difference is that the latter is under some kind of control. Either it is the 'built-in' control of the suicide pathway of differentiation – as in the transit population – or the specific feedback control of population size, as in the stem types of cell populations. Apart from that, the rest of the growth processes and cell division occur almost normally in the tumours.

The term 'almost' denotes some small, but nevertheless very important, differences from normal. One difference is that some disorders in the actual process of cell division manage to accumulate biological errors in the tumour cells. The most obvious error, which can be seen even in the microscope, shows up as chromosome abnormalities. These may vary from a simple numerical disorder, i.e. less than 46 or more than 46 chromosomes, to gross disorders with not only many more than 46 chromosomes but with some abnormally-shaped chromosomes among them (see Frontispiece).

It was said earlier in this chapter that the DNA in the chromosomes contains and conveys all the information – the genetic message – which enables the cell to express its biochemical self. If the distribution of DNA between the two daughter cells is not equal, because some error allows some extra chromosomal material to accumulate in some cells while it is missing in others then the cells become imbalanced. Most such imbalanced cells cannot live for long. The very many complex biochemical events in the cells have to be very accurately balanced to enable the cell to live. A slight degree of imbalance is usually sufficient to result in the building up of a vicious circle of metabolic abnormalities leading to cell death.

In normal cells the controlling mechanisms are tight with little or no 'tolerance'. Within the tumour cell populations, however, there is no growth control and also no efficient mechanisms for the elimination of slightly-changed cells.

One of the results of the presence of such imbalanced cells in the tumour population is that although there is no growth control, and the tumour grows, the growth is slower than it should be, because of a certain degree of cell death. In other words, as the cells divide, a certain proportion of the new cells will have new 'mistakes' or 'faults' in them, and many of these will die.

45

WHAT WE KNOW ABOUT CANCER

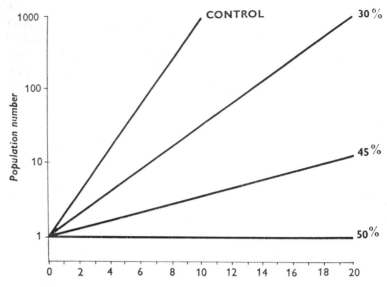

FIGURE 6

Illustration of random death slowing cell population growth. The control population with no cell death reaches the size of 1,000 cells in 10 cell cycle times. With 30 per cent random death per cell cycle, it will take 20 cell cycle times to reach the same population size, and with 50 per cent random death per cell cycle the population does not grow, it remains the same size.

This continuous cell death is a characteristic feature of most tumours. It results in a slower growth rate of the cells than would be the case without such a 'random cell death'. It must be appreciated that if the tumour cells divided (in a particular tumour) once a day, then in ten days the volume or mass of that tumour would increase one-thousandfold. With random death the slowing of the tumour growth is very considerable, as illustrated in Figure 6.

It is the popular belief that 'cancer grows faster than normal tissue cells'. This is a fallacy. Most tumours grow more slowly than normal tissues *can* grow. However, normal tissues do not grow, they maintain a steady number of their cells. In many normal tissues this is achieved without much proliferation because there is not much cell loss (e.g. liver). In other normal tissues this is achieved by maintaining a fast rate of cell division which, however, balances a fast rate of cell loss (e.g. bone marrow).

46

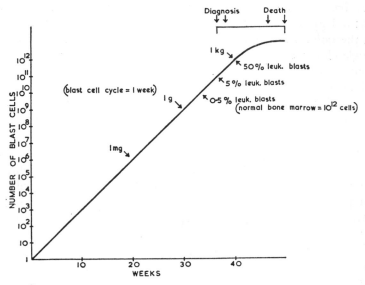

FIGURE 7

Growth of a theoretical leukaemic blast cell population. Since the normal bone marrow contains more than 1 kg. of cells (more than 10^{12}) it will take almost 40 population doublings before the leukaemia can be properly diagnosed.

Nevertheless neither the liver, nor the bone marrow *grows* in the adult organism. They are both maintained in the steady state. If and when there is a demand for growth in the liver, for example, after surgical resection of a part of it; or in the bone marrow, for example, after some toxic damage to it; then both these organs can grow back to normal population size, and they will do it faster than any cancer tissue can ever grow in size.

But there is no need for cancer to grow fast. It is enough that it is not kept in a steady state and therefore it will accumulate. Any slow growth in numbers will outgrow eventually every steady state normal cell population. And this is exactly what happens with cancer. It grows, very slowly compared with normal tissues when they grow, but since normal tissues do not grow, even the slowly-growing tumour will eventually outgrow them.

To illustrate the situation we may look at a theoretical growth curve of a leukaemic cell population (Figure 7). Assuming, for the sake of agreement, that the leukaemic cells can double their

47

number once every week, then thirty weeks will go past before about 1 gramme (approximately 1,000,000,000 cells) accumulate in the bone marrow. However, leukaemic cells do not grow in a single clump but diffusely throughout the marrow which usually contains over 1 kg. of cells (more than one million million cells). The leukaemic population is then only 1/1000 of the normal cell population – it is undetectable. Another ten doublings, however, would bring the leukaemic population also to 1 kg. By that time it is detectable, and if the patient is not treated, this number of cells will kill him. In other words by the time we can diagnose leukaemia, it has undergone at least thirty-five population doublings and if it can double five to seven times more it will kill the patient. Since we cannot hope to kill all leukaemic cells in the patient, the present treatments aim to keep the number of these cells low enough to allow continuation of the normal bone marrow function. In the future, of course, we may develop treatments that will allow a radical elimination of all leukaemic cells from the body.

II CHANGES OF NORMAL FUNCTIONS IN CANCER CELLS

The changes in cancer cells compared with normal cells can be grouped into two main categories : loss of some normal property and acquisition of some new 'abnormal' property.

However, the 'properties' of the cells which we can observe are usually the end results of very complicated chains of biochemical reactions. Therefore a 'loss' or 'gain' of some cellular function does not mean necessarily a primary loss or gain of genetic information, i.e. DNA.

It has been mentioned in the foregoing, that genetic information 'locked' in DNA can be repressed or de-repressed. Indeed, the whole process of cell differentiation in an organism is governed by a complex series of gene repressions and de-repressions.

Since cancer cells 'breed true', i.e. all descendants of a cancer cell are cancer cells of the same type, it is clear that the carcinogenic stimuli, irrespective of their nature, induce in some way, some permanent change in the genetic apparatus of the cell. Figure 8 indicates – in a very simplified way – how such changes may result in loss of growth control and also in other changes in the cell. As illustrated, changes in genes, *a*, *b* or *c*, can either inhibit another gene which inhibits the action of a latent virus, or inhibit the controlling genes which regulate when a cell should not grow, or neutralize the 'signal' which informs the controlling genes that no further growth is required. The changes in genes,

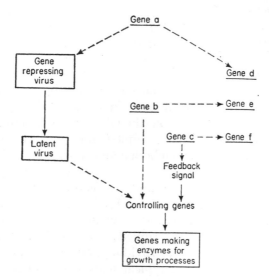

FIGURE 8

Possible ways in which genetic changes may result in uncontrolled growth. If gene a is affected it may repress another gene which normally keeps a carcinogenic virus controlled. If this gene is repressed, the virus will not be repressed and *it* may repress genes which control growth processes. Alteration in gene b may repress the controlling gene directly, and alteration in gene c may modify or inactivate the feedback 'signal' which controls the cell population size. Any of these altered genes may affect other genes (d, e, f) resulting in disturbance of other cell functions also.

a, *b* or *c*, may also influence other genes (*d*, *e* or *f*) which therefore may not function, or do so in an abnormal fashion.

It is important to realize that this is a grossly simplified scheme, and that most carcinogenic stimuli may induce direct or indirect changes in many genes simultaneously. This of course will complicate the picture considerably and will result in a wide spectrum of changes within the cells.

Most cells, where genetic apparatus is interfered with in a non-specific way will die eventually. Since we do not possess any way in which specific changes in the genome can be produced by chemicals (directly or indirectly) the few cells surviving non-specific genetic damage may show wide differences from each other.

(a) Contact inhibition

If normal cells are explanted from the body into a suitable nutrient medium in glass or plastic containers, they can start to proliferate. As the cells multiply, they will occupy an increasingly larger proportion of the available solid surface (glass or plastic), This 'occupation' will be achieved not only by mere numerical increase, but will be facilitated – in certain cell types – by the active movement of cells on the glass surface. When all the available surface has been occupied, and the cells are in full contact with each other, then both active movement and proliferation will cease. This is called contact inhibition of movement and contact inhibition of growth, and is a feature of normal cells.

Cancer cells have lost this normal function. If explanted into a glass vessel, they will grow and move around even when all the available glass surface is occupied; they will crawl on top of each other and will continue dividing also for a while. This 'loss of contact inhibition' is a typical feature of cancer cells. One must point out, however, that this is not an all or none feature; in other words it is not true to say that all normal cells have complete contact inhibition and all cancer cells have no contact inhibition whatever. The difference between normal cells and cancer cells, in that respect, is more of quantity than of quality. There are some normal cell types which tend to crawl over each other, and there are some cancer cells which tend to slow their growth and movement when in close contact with each other. However, the difference by and large is a typical feature of malignant cells.

The nature and mechanism of contact inhibition is not fully understood. It probably depends on some property of the cell's surface, the cell membrane. It is also thought to be involved in the normal 'recognition of self' since if two different types of normal cells are explanted, they may not show contact inhibition on meeting each other. In these culture conditions, the normal cells may have to recognize each other's 'self' to exhibit contact inhibition.

The characteristic difference between a 'benign' tumour and cancer is that cancer can invade the neighbouring tissues, while the 'benign' tumour remains well demarcated from the surrounding normal tissue. Also, cancer cells can spread to distant body sites, to produce 'secondary deposits' or 'distant metastases'. The benign tumours do not produce such distant spread. It is tempting to correlate the loss of contact inhibition with the capacity of the cells to invade surrounding normal tissue and also with the ability to settle down in distant parts of the body. However, this is not likely to be a good explanation since two different normal tissues may not show contact inhibition to each other, and there are many normal cells (the white blood cells in particular) which can infiltrate any normal tissue, and can travel with the blood to any site in the body, where they can 'settle down'. Indeed, without this infiltrating and travelling ability of the normal white blood cells, the body could not combat bacterial infections.

(b) Biochemical functions
Throughout the last three decades a vast amount of work has been devoted to finding out what the basic biochemical difference is between normal and cancerous cells. Clearly, if one understood or found some essential difference, it could be exploited for the treatment of cancer. It can be fairly stated that there is no property or biochemical function which has not been investigated both in normal and in malignant cells. Published work on these investigations would fill many volumes. Since new biochemical techniques are being developed constantly, this type of work is continuing in the hope that some exploitable difference will be found eventually.

At present, however, there is no evidence for the absence or presence of any biochemical function which would be characteristic for cancer cells. The summary of findings in this respect is that most cancer cells are slightly deficient in some of the enzymes which the normal cells possess. This statement is, of course, a broad generalization, since there are great differences between different normal cells. Nevertheless, by and large, cancer cells tend to be less efficient in most biochemical functions than normal cells. Most, but not all. There are some functions, for example, the ability to exist without much oxygen, in respect of which most cancer cells are more efficient than most normal cells.

51

Loss of differentiation is a common feature of cancer cells. To take two examples : normal breast gland or normal thyroid gland have not only well-recognizable morphological features which can be identified under the microscope, but they also have characteristic biochemical features. In the breast gland these manifest themselves in the response to certain hormones, and in the thyroid gland in the production of the hormone, thyroxin.

In cancer of the breast and in cancer of the thyroid, even in the very earliest stages of the disease, there will be recognizable deficiencies in these normal functions. Nevertheless, for a while some breast cancers may respond to hormone treatment, and for a while some thyroid cancers will continue to synthesize thyroxin. With the progress of the disease, these functions will be progressively lost in the cancer cells. Similarly, normal bone-marrow stem cells will respond to certain stimuli and will produce normal red cells or white cells. However, the 'blast' cells of acute leukaemia have lost this capacity to respond to normal stimuli of differentiation – they will not make red cells or normal white cells, they will remain 'blast' cells (not very dissimilar in appearance to the normal very young bone-marrow cells) and will keep dividing as such.

It has been mentioned earlier that the cell is a very complex chemical factory with hundreds of different reactions taking place in it at any time. Many of the functions are common to all cells, these are the functions which are essential to normal cellular existence. There are other functions which are specific for certain 'differentiated' normal cells. The change from normal to cancer cell appears to involve a partial loss of these specialized chemical functions. The more basic functions however remain. The loss of specialized functions may make the cancer cells more 'resilient' in the sense that they may survive in some conditions which are too adverse for normal cells.

The most important feature of the loss of biochemical properties is a loss of 'self' of the cell. Feedback controls for growth as well as stimuli for differentiation depend on the presence of suitable apparatus within the cell, i.e. on the biochemical or physicochemical identity of the appropriate cell type. Loss of such properties from the cell result – by definition – in a change in the identity of the cell. This change of identity has far-reaching effects, and in the case of cancer cells results in some further subtle changes.

Most normal cells, if they suffer some functional loss, tend to lose their viability. Also, there is in the body an elaborate and sensitive mechanism which rejects all cells which are 'foreign' or 'non-self'. This is the well known immunological rejection phenomenon. (v.i.) The change in cancer cells is, however, such that while their 'self' is changing sufficiently not to recognize normal control, it is not changing sufficiently to elicit an effective rejection reaction from the immune system of the body.

This does not mean that cancer cells are not recognized by the body as 'foreign'. In many, perhaps in most instances, they are eliciting some immune reaction, and this immune reaction contributes to the random death rate occurring among cancer cells. Also, in some instances, this immune reaction may assist in eliminating cancer cells after drug therapy (for example, in choriocarcinoma of women). Nevertheless, there is a sufficient loss of 'antigenicity' (i.e. capacity to elicit an immune reaction) in cancer cells to enable them to exist and grow in spite of their relative foreignness in the body.

To summarize therefore, the cancer cells tend to resemble the normal cell types from which they originated, and in some respects there is more resemblance between a normal cell and its cancerous derivative than between two different types of cancer cells. However, with advancing malignancy the tumour cells tend to become more 'primitive' and resemble each other more than any normal cell type. Finally, much of the changes observed during carcinogenesis appear to be losses of properties and functions rather than development of 'new' properties.

CONCLUSIONS

Although by necessity greatly simplified, the foregoing attempts to illustrate the present state of knowledge about the nature of cancer. It is clear that our knowledge in this respect is inadequate, in spite of the very great amount of effort which has been expended by so many investigators in numerous laboratories. When it comes to define cancer or malignant growth of any kind, we can still only speak in generalities : loss of growth control, loss of power to differentiate, loss of various enzyme functions, loss of contact inhibition, loss of antigenicity, and so on. These losses are, furthermore, rarely absolute. Some vestige of growth control, of a kind, exists in some tumours, some degree of differentiation exists in many. The real question : the essential difference between normal and cancer cell is still not known in precise biochemical or physicochemical terms.

In retrospect, we know now that the essential difference between normal and cancerous cells lies in some aspect of the genetic code of the cell – structurally or functionally. It is only now, during the last few years, that methods have become available for the study of the fine structure of the genetic code. Most of the techniques available still only apply to micro-organisms or viruses, and considerable methodological improvement is necessary before the same resolution could be expected with the much more complex mammalian cells.

It has been said many times that cancer research follows three main directions : the study of the cause, the nature and the cure of cancer. After five decades of intensive work by hundreds of scientists it appears that these three lines approach each other closely in the study of the molecular biology of cancer. The understanding of the molecular events in the various steps in carcinogenesis, the molecular events specific for cancer cells, and the molecular events with various new drugs hopefully designed for the purpose, is the aim towards which modern cancer research is going. The understanding of the nature of cancer, in molecular terms, is the necessary prerequisite for rational attempts at new treatment design. Attempts at 'short cuts' will be and should be made; there is always a demand in science for inspired guessing. However, the steady and increasing erosion of the problem of cancer will depend on the understanding of the basic mechanisms involved.

CHAPTER III

THE HISTORY OF CANCER RESEARCH

R. J. C. HARRIS

THE FATEFUL DECADE

The seminal period in the history of cancer research was, without doubt, the eleven years between 1905 and 1915. In 1902 the Imperial Cancer Research Fund had been founded in London and the first director, E. F. Bashford, had proposed a scheme of research and had, himself, begun studies on the biological and morphological properties of spontaneous and transmissible mouse tumours. By 1906 B. Fischer was investigating cancer-production

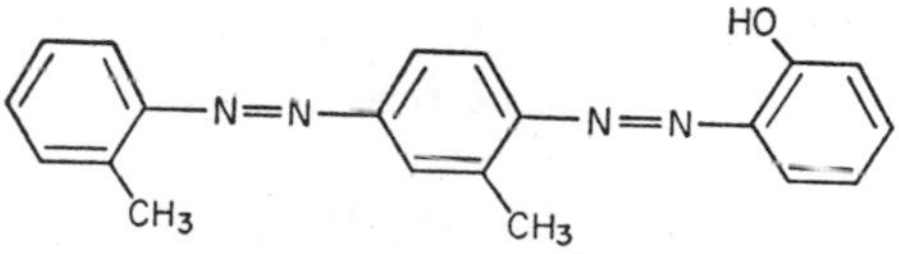

FIGURE 9 'Scarlet red'

by azo dyes such as 'scarlet red' after inoculating the substance into the skin of a rabbit's ear.

The early years of this twentieth century also saw a change of perspective so far as coal-tar cancers were concerned. Originally it was believed that these cancers were caused by mechanical injury (irritation – v.) but now they became associated with chemical injury and Ross and Cropper suggested in 1911 that chemical substances in the tar or pitch directly induced cell division. Yamagiwa and Ichikawa in 1915 were the first to succeed in inducing tumours in the ears of rabbits by persistent application of tar. Meanwhile, in 1908, Ellerman and Bang had transmitted chicken leukosis to chicks with extracts of the malignant tissue which did not contain living cells (cell-free extracts). However, at this time leukosis was not considered to be a

55

malignant condition and to Rous in 1911 is attributed the discovery of the first cancer-producing virus, that of chicken sarcoma.

X-rays were first discovered by Roentgen in 1895 and by 1896 the first case of radiation-induced dermatitis had appeared. In 1902 Frieben described a cancer in a 33 year-old technician who, for four years only, had demonstrated X-ray techniques. Within twelve years, Feygin had collected 104 cases from the literature and, since that time, more than 1,000 cases have been recorded. For X-radiation the human 'experiment' came first as, indeed, it had for tar and soot, but Clunet in 1910 succeeded in inducing sarcomas in two irradiated rats after latent periods of nine months and two years respectively.

In this short period, carcinogenic (cancer-producing) potentiality had been shown for three quite different types of agency — physical (X-radiation), chemical (tar, azo dyes) and biological (viruses).

THE PROPHETIC SCOTS

Of course, these important discoveries did not arrive unheralded — in fact the direction of cancer research had been prophetically discovered by a handful of Scottish physicians and surgeons (the Medical Committee of the Society for Investigating the Nature and Cure of Cancer) in 1802. They published their report in the *Edinburgh Medical and Surgical Journal* of 1806 (vol. 2, pp. 382-9).

Before them they would have had at least two important works on the causes of cancer — both published in 1775. In the first, Percival Pott (better known, perhaps, for Pott's fracture) described a particular form of skin cancer, scrotal epithelioma, in chimney sweeps. Pott ascribed this — the first occupational cancer — to a specific cause : namely, continuous exposure of the skin to soot. In those days chimney sweeps began as 'climbing boys' and it was, said Pott, this long exposure to soot which caused the cancers. In that same year the Academy of Sciences at Lyons offered a prize for the best essay on the causes of cancer. The prize was won by Peyrilhe who described his successful experiments in transplanting cancer from man into dogs. In fact, Peyrilhe had not succeeded in this. The 'cancer' in the dog was certainly a tumour (swelling) but it was composed of disintegrating human tissue together with those cells and fluids from the dog which were actively engaged in trying to remove the foreign (and, no doubt, infected) tissue. That such a mistake could be made by such a learned body is attributable to the fact that no one, at that time, knew anything about the structure and cellularity of tumours, or the nature of bacterial infections.

In the light of this (and the implied criticism of Pott's work in Query 8) the Scottish queries, and comments on the queries (which I have shortened from the original), are outstanding. So much so that 166 years later we only have partial answers to some of the questions.

THE SCOTTISH QUESTIONNAIRE

QUERY 1: *What are the diagnostic signs of cancer?*

It is very much to be wished that we had an exact definition of cancer, those of the nosologists [nosology is the classification of disease] being very imperfect and insufficient. It has accordingly happened that a disease, which has been denominated cancer by one medical man, has not been allowed to be such by another; and painful and hazardous operations have been performed by some, which were not thought necessary. . . . If a just and exact definition of cancer cannot yet be formed, we must be satisfied with such a description as a correct history of the disease will afford.

QUERY 2: *Does any alteration in the structure of a part take place, preceding that more obvious change which is called cancer; and if there be an alteration, what is its nature?*

It might first be asked, does any disposition to cancer in any part take place previously to any physical alteration or change of structure in the part? or are there any symptoms, local or constitutional, which denote that cancer is about to be formed? Then we may consider how the first alteration in the structure of a part, disposed to become cancerous, is to be distinguished from the structure of parts disposed to other diseases.

. . . One great consequence of obtaining an answer to this query would be, that though we are unable to cure cancer in an

57

advanced stage, we might extinguish the disposition to it, or suppress it completely in an early stage, whether the disposition or the progress consist in increased or new action of a part, or in a change of structure.

QUERY 3: *Is cancer always an original and primary disease; or may other diseases degenerate into cancer?*

This is a question which has been very much disputed; at least there have been many different opinions concerning it. It does not imply that all the changes which take place from the commencement of the same disease, through its progress to the time when it is acknowledged to be indubitably a disease of a certain kind, should bear an exact or close resemblance : but it relates to the absolute change in the essence of one disease to that of another, with which it had originally no resemblance or affinity. We must, therefore, leave this query to be determined by future experience and observation.

QUERY 4: *Are there any proofs of cancer being an hereditary disease?*

Whether cancer or any other disease be, strictly speaking, hereditary, has, like many other opinions, been positively asserted, and as positively denied. Whether children born of cancerous parents be more liable to cancer than others, from any structure or organization of the body, or any rooted principle of the constitution, may, by attentive observation, be discovered; and, if it should be so proved, we might be led to the prevention of cancer by medicine, by well-regulated diet, or a circumspect manner of education, and of living. If it be proved, on the contrary, that cancer is not hereditary, the minds of many would be relieved from the distress of perpetual apprehension.

QUERY 5: *Are there any proofs of cancer being a contagious disease?*

This query certainly requires some explanation. Does it imply a possibility of cancer being conveyed from one person to another by the breath, as in the hooping-cough, and, as some have suspected, in consumption? or by effluvia exhaled from a body afflicted with this disease, as in infectious fevers? or by the breath passing over an ulcerated surface, as in cancer of the mouth or lip? The opinion of cancer being contagious having been advanced, it is become necessary to discuss it, as far as we can, by observation, by experiments, and by casual occurrences.

QUERY 6: *Is there any well-marked relation between cancer and other diseases? If there be, what are those diseases to which it bears the nearest resemblance in its origin, progress, and termination?*

Whether there be any relation or affinity between cancer and other diseases acknowledged not to be cancerous, as is the case with all unproved assertions, has been by some affirmed, and by others denied. The second part of this query is equally supported and maintained. Some have been assured of the affinity between cancer and scrophula, and others of that between cancer and syphilis; but neither of these opinions have been proved or well supported by a just statement of facts, by regular induction, nor by any collateral circumstance accompanying methods of cure, or the use of any particular medicine. Is it proved that cancer of the breast is exactly the same disease as cancer of the tongue, or that of the uterus? or that, in every case of cancer, in any part, the same method of treatment will be proper? The distinction of similar diseases, is very necessary, because medicines, which may be of service in one of these, may be injurious in another. Let us hope that, when precise distinctions are made between cancer and resembling diseases, and between the various kinds of cancer, appropriate and efficacious methods of treatment of each disease will follow to the great benefit and relief of the afflicted, and to the credit of the profession.

QUERY 7: *May cancer be regarded at any period, or under any circumstances, merely as a local disease? Or does the existence of cancer in one part afford a presumption that there is a tendency to a similar morbid alteration in other parts of the animal system?*

An answer to this query would be highly important, as it is the *experimentum crucis* of many operations which have been performed for the extirpation of cancerous parts. In cancer of one part, perhaps, all similar and sympathizing parts may be

59

affected; perhaps the whole constitution. A surgeon, who is said to have great skill and success in removing cancerous breasts, has said, that in many truly cancerous affections of that part, he had found, on examination, that the uterus exhibited marks of the same disease, and that the state of the uterus was his guide in determining him to extirpate or to avoid operating upon diseased breasts. If the uterus was discovered to be affected, he refused to perform the operation, having constantly found it unsuccessful under such circumstances; yet it does not follow that all extirpations of the breast will be successful, if the uterus be free from disease. When operations fail to remove the whole disease, which is in some cases impracticable, the sufferings of the patients are aggravated, and their lives shortened, by operations; of course they ought not then to be performed. Tumours in the breast, of a considerable size, will often remain in a quiescent state for many years, even to the close of life, if not disturbed by injudicious treatment or extraneous injuries, of which the ancients were well aware. It therefore appears as improper to extirpate these as it does to suffer them to remain, when they begin to be disturbed, and can be wholly removed. It appears that more caution than has been usually exercised seems necessary in these operations. It is also requisite to decide, by repeated trials, whether the extirpation of cancerous breasts by the knife or caustic be preferable, as far as relates to the operation, or a prospect of a return of the disease. In practice, we must distinguish between the extirpation of a diseased part and the cure of the disease; the latter of which is the object of these queries, as many parts which do not admit of extirpation are liable to cancer.

QUERY 8: *Has climate or local situation any influence in rendering the human constitution more or less liable to cancer, under any form, or in any part?*

There is a considerable variety in the disease to which human beings are liable in hot and cold climates, and in damp or dry situations, or in those which are low or exposed. The Goitre has not been found, or very rarely, in warm and flat countries, nor the Yaws in cold ones. The Lepra, of every kind, is infinitely more frequent in some countries than in others, and more virulent. With regard to cancer, it is not only necessary to observe the effects of climate and local situation, but to extend our views to different employments, as those in various metals and manufactures; in mines and collieries; in the army and navy; in those who lead sedentary or active lives; in the married or single; in the different sexes, and many other circumstances. Should it be proved that women are more subject to cancer than men, we may then inquire whether married women are more liable to have the uterus or breasts affected; those who have had children or not; those who have suckled, or those who did not; and the same observations may be made of the single. The cancer to which chimney-sweepers are subject is known, but not accurately understood; and none but fruitless observations have yet been made upon it, except such as relate to operations.

QUERY 9: *Is there any particular temperament of body more liable to be affected with cancer than others? If there be, what is the nature of that temperament?*

The word temperament has been often used by medical writers without any precise meaning. It is here meant to signify any native or acquired habit of body, which may dispose to, or resist, the influence of cancer. Should this query be answered in the affirmative, having discovered the temperament most liable to cancer, we might be led to the prevention of this disease, as was before observed under query 4.

QUERY 10: *Are brute creatures subject to any disease resembling cancer in the human body?*

It is not at present known whether brute creatures are subject to cancer, though some of their diseases have a very suspicious appearance. When this question is decided, we may inquire what class of animals is chiefly subjected to cancer; the wild or the domesticated; the carniverous or the graminivorous; those which do, or those which do not, chew the cud. This investigation may lead to much philosophical amusement and useful information; particularly it may teach us how far the prevalence or frequency of cancer may depend upon the manners and habits of life. As establishments are now formed for the reception of several kinds of animals, and, as the treatment of their diseases has at length fallen under the care of scientific men, it is hoped that the information here required may be readily obtained. If animals

61

which live only on herbs, and never drink any other liquid than water, prove to be the least, or not at all, subject to cancer, such proof may, in many cases, become a guide in practice.

QUERY 11 : *Is there any period of life absolutely exempt from the attack of this disease?*

With regard to the periods of life when human beings are most or at all liable to cancer, it seems to be generally admitted to be most frequent in old or advanced in age; but this is not satisfactorily proved. Nor is it certainly known what is the earliest period of life at which cancer has been observed to take place; though no case of that disease has yet been noticed before twenty years of age; at least not before the time of puberty, when the parts, most frequently affected with cancer, undergo a great and conspicuous change, so that some connexion may possibly be observed between puberty and this disease. The same may also perhaps be observed at the time of the final cessation of the menses. Among large bodies of children collected together in charity and other schools, or of adults in hospitals, in convents, and in monasteries, opportunities of answering this question must certainly occur.

QUERY 12 : *Are the lymphatic glands ever affected primarily in this disease?*

This query goes to the very root of inquiry with respect to cancer, which has been hitherto said always to originate in the glandular system, without distinguishing, however, the particular set of glands. In cancerous affections of the eye, it is believed that the ball of the eye is not primarily affected, but the lachrymal gland. In cancers of the breast, the lymphatic glands appear to be affected only in a secondary way, when the disease is making progress. It is probable that careful attention to the objects of this query would lead to many new observations respecting the first seat, cause, and effect of cancer.

QUERY 13 : *Is cancer, under any circumstances, susceptible of a natural cure?*

Many diseases and accidents, to which the human body is liable, are cured or repaired by some process of the constitution peculiarly and admirably adapted to the kind of disease or accident. The principle of this process, or the process itself, has usually been expressed by the term Nature, and, in medical language, more frequently *Vis Medicatrix*. But no instance has ever occurred, or been recorded, of cancer being cured by any natural process of the constitution. . . . Facts alone, and those indubitably proved, are in this place to be admitted, till such a number shall be collected as will enable us to establish, by fair induction, a sound practice, no longer the creature of presumption or vain opinions.

AETIOLOGICAL HYPOTHESES

The relevance of these queries and comments is all the more remarkable when one considers that 'cell-theory' was still fifty years or so away from acceptance. Hooke in 1665 had espied 'cellules' in cork bark and similar structures were accepted as the elementary units of all living matter by 1855 (Virchow — *omnis cellula e cellula*). Cancers, too, were found to be composed of cells. How the cells of cancers related to the other cells of the body was the subject of two rival theories, and three hypotheses to account for the change of the one into the other. The first theory stated that any normal cell still capable of multiplying could become cancerous, but the second theory postulated that cancers arose from abnormal cells within the normal tissue populations.

The first hypothesis related malignant change to chronic irritation of tissues, leading to inflammation and then to cancer. It was based on observation because it was well attested that cancers could arise in scars, ulcerations and fistulae in the skin. Cancers arising from continuous sunburn, X-irradiation, burns, industrial exposure to tar or betel-nut chewing, were all accepted as evidence for this hypothesis.

As the sole hypothesis, however, it ran into difficulties (as, indeed, do all single hypotheses for the cause of cancer). Thus, not all conditions of pre-malignancy produced by irritative agents go on to full malignancy, and some forms of cancer never arise in this way.

The second hypothesis relates to the second theory. Lobstein and Récamier (1829) noticed (as had others) that the cells of some cancers bore a striking resemblance to cells of embryonic tissues.

They supposed, therefore, that cancers arose by the multiplication of embryonic cells of the individual which had somehow persisted in the adult structure of the organism. Such 'embryonal nests' are certainly to be found in nearly all tissues and organs – so many of them, in fact, that the great majority could never become malignant. Cohnheim combined this hypothesis with that of irritation but there is no present evidence for selecting out particular cell populations in this way.

The third hypothesis is that parasites cause cancer and, in the sense that viruses are parasites, this hypothesis is still valid. However, towards the end of the nineteenth century, pathologists were taking advantage of Pasteur's discovery of microbes as causes of disease and 'finding' them as causes as cancer. In 1896 Rappini discovered his 'diplococcus' and in 1901 Royen isolated 'micrococcus neoformans' from cancers – apparently a common-or-garden staphylococcus. The fact that doctors and nurses in close contact with patients with cancer do not contract the disease preferentially seems to dispose of cancer as a contagious disease, but viruses may pose different problems which we shall consider later.

TRANSPLANTABLE ANIMAL TUMOURS

It was realized as early as 1806 that the question of cancer in animals might well be important for the light that might be shed on the disease in man. Cancers were soon discovered in mammals, especially rats and mice, and in birds (although there was some dispute about the exact nature of the virus-induced growths studied by Rous and his colleagues). In general they occurred but rarely in early laboratory stocks of animals and it soon became apparent that, in order to study them more easily, a way of transplanting them from animal to animal should be sought. For many years following Peyrilhe's prize award, methods were sought for transplanting tumours from man into animals – without, of course, any conclusive results. The first real observation of value was the successful transplantation by Klencke in 1843 of a melanotic tumour of the eye of a horse into the eye of another horse. The most probable reason why this was successful was quite unknown to Klencke. The eye is an immunologically privileged site and the forces of tissue rejection which operate so infallibly elsewhere in the body are weaker, or non-existent, at this site. Rudnev, at St Petersburg in 1870, laid the first ground rules for successful tumour transplantation. First, use living cells from the donor's tumour; second, use a host animal of the same species; third, use small pieces of tissue and fourth, use young animals. Following the rules of his professor, one of Rudnev's pupils, Novinskii, succeeded in 1877 in transplanting three dog tumours into puppies and this paper is generally agreed to herald the success of tumour transplantation.

HOST RESISTANCE TO TRANSPLANTATION

However, in the early years of this century those who were working with transplanted mouse or rat tumours soon noticed that not all the grafts grew, even though they had been made under apparently identical conditions. This was correctly ascribed to differences in the resistance of the host animals. Animals in which the grafts did not grow, or from which they disappeared after limited growth, were apparently resistant to further grafts of the same tumour. There was an immediate hope that a study of the nature of this resistance might lead to methods for preventing or treating cancer in man. It was soon discovered, however, that resistance to tumour grafts could equally well be brought about by inoculating normal tissue from the donor into the host. The resistance so induced had no effect on the growth of an existing *spontaneous* tumour, or, indeed, on the animal's chances of later developing one. This was the general resistance of one animal to the tissues of another (except its identical twin) with which we are today so familiar in grafting organs from one human individual to another.

The exception to this resistance phenomenon was discovered by Tyzzer in 1907. He found that spontaneous tumours in Japanese waltzing mice could always be successfully transplanted into other waltzing mice. In non-waltzing mice the tumour transplants failed to grow. The reason lay in the fact that the breeding of the waltzing mice had to be carefully controlled so that the offspring retained the waltzing characteristic. This degree of required in-breeding resulted in such a genetic homogeneity that the tissues of one animal were no more foreign to another than those of one identical twin to the other. The secret of tumour transplantation – as, indeed, of all successful tissue transplantation – was genetic homogeneity. The properties of transplanted animal tumours still engage the interests of many in cancer research and every laboratory will have its different strains of inbred (brother mated to sister) rats and mice. Many of these laboratories will be carrying, by serial transplantation, tumours which first arose in rats or mice tens of years before—what these tumours, themselves, are carrying is another story which we shall consider later! Moreover, the incidence of spontaneous cancer varies greatly between these different strains. Some mice have a very high incidence of breast cancer, and others a high incidence of leukaemia. Some are especially prone to develop benign lung tumours and yet others have a genetic resistance to lung tumours. The use of such animals for the study of the origin of different forms of cancer is obvious.

THE EXPERIMENTAL PRODUCTION OF CANCER

Percival Pott described scrotal epithelioma as an occupational cancer of chimney-sweeps in 1775, but it was only a hundred years later in 1875 that von Volkmann discovered occupational skin cancers among workers in the tar and paraffin industry at Halle and, in 1876, Joseph Bell described similar cases among Scottish shale-oil workers. In 1887 operatives in the Lancashire cotton-spinning mills were found to suffer from similar skin cancers and these are now known to have been a result of prolonged contact with the mineral oils used to lubricate the machinery. It is scandalous that, even today, lubricating oils containing cancer-producing chemical compounds (carcinogens) are still being used in some industries in this, and other countries.

The 'occupational' skin cancers all pointed to a possible source of carcinogens which could be used in systematic animal experiments and, as we have already noted, Yamagiwa and Ichikawa succeeded, in 1915, in inducing tumours in the ears of rabbits by long application of coal-tar. In 1922, R. D. Passey showed that soot was carcinogenic and the drive then began to isolate the actual substance(s) responsible.

THE FRACTIONATION OF COAL TAR

Bloch and Dreifus in Zürich in 1921 provided the first clue. They found that the carcinogen(s) contained carbon and hydrogen, but not nitrogen, sulphur or arsenic and deduced that they were probably complex (polycyclic) hydrocarbons based on benzene. Sir Ernest Kennaway, at the Royal Cancer Hospital in London, was able to produce carcinogenic 'tars' by heating a number of natural products (such as cholesterol, yeast or human hair) to high temperatures in the presence of hydrogen gas. Mayneord investigating a blue fluorescence always present when the tars were carcinogenic, found in 1927 that this fluorescence spectrum was characteristic. There was thus a 'thin blue line' with which to thread through the chemical maze of the carcinogenic tars and oils. Hieger, in 1928, noticed that 1 : 2-benzanthracene had so similar a fluorescence spectrum as to leave no doubt that some substance similar to it, and probably a derivative of it, was responsible for the thin blue line that linked the cancer production to a chemical.

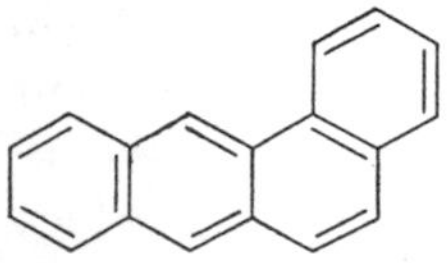

FIGURE 10   1 : 2-benzanthracene

Clar, in 1930, made the more complex, but related 1 : 2 : 5 : 6-dibenzanthracene and this became the first *pure* chemical compound to be shown to be cancer-producing (Kennaway and Hieger, 1930).

The data were now at hand for an attack on the tars and the

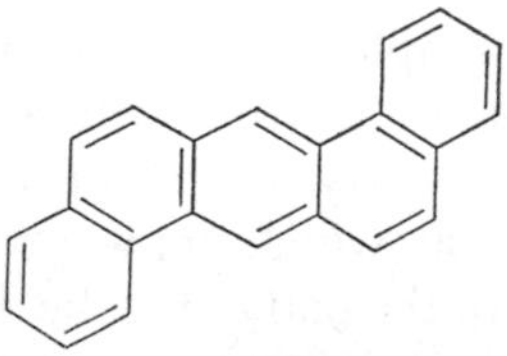

FIGURE 11   1 : 2 : 5 : 6-dibenzanthracene

Royal Cancer Hospital team began the fractionation of two tons of pitch from Becton gas-works. By the autumn of 1931 this had been reduced to 7 grammes of a yellow crystalline powder. The major component of this, 3 : 4-benzpyrene, was, as predicted, a carcinogenic polycyclic hydrocarbon related to 1 : 2-benzanthracene, and showing the strong blue fluorescence of the original pitch.

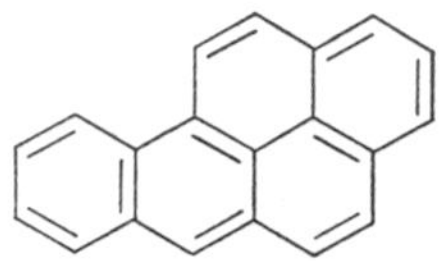

FIGURE 12   3 : 4-benzpyrene

The solution to the problem of the causes of cancer now seemed very close to hand and the search began in laboratories the world over, for pure chemical compounds with similar cancer-producing properties; very many are now known. No doubt the carcinogenic polycyclic hydrocarbons in tars and mineral oils are responsible for the occupational cancers which have occurred in those exposed to them. Many of the complex steroid hormones, and cholesterol, which occur in the animal body have chemical structures which superficially resemble those of the polycyclic hydrocarbons, but no one has yet shown that the body can convert the steroids to known carcinogenic hydrocarbons or, conversely, can build up a carcinogen instead of the normal product.

CHEMICAL CARCINOGENS

These complex chemicals exert their influence mainly at the site of application, for example, the skin of man or animal. Other sorts of carcinogen (and there are now many hundreds of chemical substances with this property) act at sites remote from the point of application – points at which some product of the chemical, after its interaction with the body, may be deposited.

Fischer, in 1906, had injected 'scarlet red' dye (see p. 55) into the skin of the rabbits' ear and had produced tumour-like masses. In 1909 Hayward found that a portion of this structure (4'-amino – 2 : 3'-azotoluene) was carcinogenic.

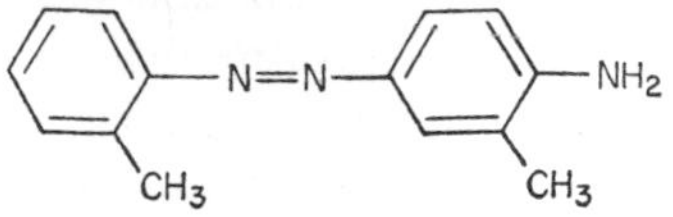

FIGURE 13

But when this was fed to rats (rather than injected) over a long period they contracted liver cancer. In 1936 Riojun Kinosita fed an orange dye 'butter-yellow' to rats and found that this was most effective as a liver carcinogen.

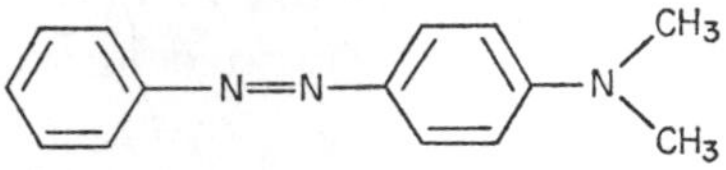

FIGURE 14 4-dimethylaminoazobenzene ('butter-yellow')

There can be little doubt that Kinosita's discovery prevented this dye from being used as a colouring agent for butter!

OCCUPATIONAL BLADDER CANCER

Just as the study of occupational skin cancer led to the discovery of the polycyclic hydrocarbon carcinogens, occupational bladder cancer in the chemical (dyestuffs) industry uncovered a new group of carcinogenic compounds (the aromatic amines – Figure 15).

There is a small 'spontaneous' incidence of bladder cancer in the general population but the risk was more than thirty times greater in some chemical workers and the average age of onset was some fifteen years earlier. The chemical substances involved are principally β-naphthylamine (2-naphthylamine) and benzidine. Rehn, in 1895, thought that aniline was the cause because he had noted bladder cancer in aniline dye workers.

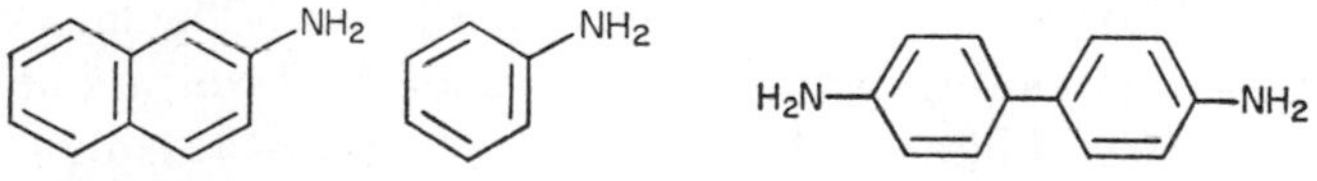

2-naphthylamine   aniline   benzidine

FIGURE 15

69

The risk of occupational bladder cancer was also known in the rubber industries—associated with the manufacture of tyres and heavy electric cables. The induction period for the disease is about fifteen to twenty years and analysis of cases suggests that the hazard first became apparent in rubber works in 1928 when an anti-oxidant (which contained about 2·5 per cent 2-naphthylamine) was used in rubber compounding.

With universal knowledge of the dangers involved, the manufacture and use of these carcinogenic amines has almost ceased.

It is pertinent to ask, of course, why these chemicals, which enter the body via the skin, the lungs, or the mouth, produce cancer in the *bladder*. Animal experiments show that, in the body, 2-naphthylamine is converted to derivatives of 2-amino-1-naphthol and it is these, concentrated in the urine, which are responsible for the cancers.

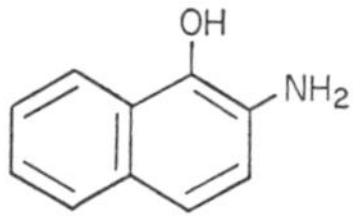

FIGURE 16   2-amino-1-naphthol

Man, dog, rat and rabbit convert 2-naphthylamine in this way, but, in the mouse, liver, and not bladder, cancers are induced. This suggests that the mouse has a different way (metabolism) of dealing with these substances.

There is nothing in the presentation of this disease to distinguish 'occupational' bladder cancers from those for which there was no exposure to 2-naphthylamine. This has led to the very interesting suggestion that the spontaneous cancers may have a similar aetiology in that some error of metabolism in the individual leads to the production of carcinogens from substances normally present in urine.

There is thus an enormous variety of chemical substances capable of converting normal cells to malignant. The lack of any chemical relationship between these has long been a stumbling block to any unitary theory of carcinogenesis—although many attempts have been made to find this, not only for chemicals but for viruses and radiation as well. One or two of the more recent theories will be discussed briefly below after a consideration of physical and viral carcinogens.

CANCER-PRODUCTION BY HORMONES

Carcinogens may possibly be produced within the human, or animal, body (endogenously) by some metabolic error (as for bladder cancer), by some aberration in the manufacture of a normal body component (such as a steroid hormone) or even by the aberrant action (perhaps because of a deficit or a surfeit) of such a hormone.

Loeb, in 1919, found that if the ovaries of mice were removed (oophorectomy) before they were four months old, such animals did not develop spontaneous breast cancer. Lacassagne developed this idea in 1932 in the opposite sense. Giving female sex hormone (oestrone) to mice (rather than removing it by removing the ovaries) increased the incidence of breast cancer in the females, and caused such a cancer in *male* mice. The male hormone, testosterone, had the same effect as oophorectomy.

Later it was shown that the synthetic female sex hormone (diethylstilboestrol) was as efficient as oestrone.

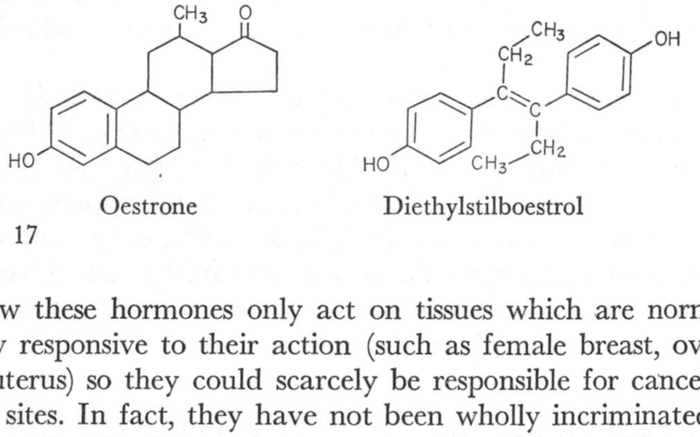

Oestrone   Diethylstilboestrol

FIGURE 17

Now these hormones only act on tissues which are normally highly responsive to their action (such as female breast, ovaries and uterus) so they could scarcely be responsible for cancers at other sites. In fact, they have not been wholly incriminated for cancers of endocrine organs in women (see Chapter IX).

CANCER PRODUCTION BY RADIATION

The induction of cancer by X-rays which, as we have already seen, was discovered during that triumphant decade at the beginning of this century, was extended to include chemical elements which liberate either gamma-rays, sub-atomic particles, or X-particles by radioactive decay. Thus, in 1924 an American dentist, Blum, found that women who had been engaged in painting instrument dials with radioactive (luminescent) paint were presenting with jaw necrosis. They customarily produced a 'tip' to the brush with their lips and had thereby ingested some of the radioactive elements in the paint, the atoms of which, after replacing calcium in the bones of the jaw, subsequently disintegrated and the radiation then liberated caused necrosis of the bones. In 1928 the first cases of sarcomas of these bones were appearing and, by 1931 nine cases had occurred with a latent period, between exposure and clinical disease, of between four and eleven years. It has since been shown that ingestion of as little as one-hundredth of a milligram of radium bromide is sufficient to cause bone cancer. Some gases, such as radon and thoron, are radioactive, and lung cancers subsequently attributable to these were seen in miners in Schneeberg. Originally these were thought by Harting and Hesse in 1879 to be caused by arsenic in the ore being mined, but miners at Joachimstahl in central Europe also contracted lung cancer. The uranium ore there was arsenic-free, but the mine air contained radon, produced by radioactive disintegration of radium salts in the ore.

Great concern has more recently been generated about radioactive 'fall-out' from atomic explosives or from effluents of atomic power stations. Fortunately, only the Chinese are currently adding to the former, and present-day precautions are minimizing the dangers from the latter. Unhappily radiation has only a very low threshold and it would be true to say that all radiation is harmful whether it comes from diagnostic X-rays or even from the fast-disappearing fluoroscopes in shoe-shops.

CANCER PRODUCTION BY PARASITES

The most significant biological, as distinct from chemical and physical, carcinogens are viruses, but even before the discovery of viruses as disease-producing organisms, animal parasites had been implicated in the induction of cancer. In 1888 Virchow concluded that 5 per cent of patients with bilharzia (a bladder disease caused by *Schistosoma haematobium*) developed bladder cancer. Today this association is no longer thought to be a simple one and other, possibly dietary, factors are known to be involved. Fibiger, between 1913 and 1920, identified a small nematode (originally called *Spiroptera*, but now known as *Congylonema neoplasticum*) in stomach cancers in wild rats. He found that the intermediate host for this parasite was the American cockroach *(Blatte americana)*. The cockroaches ate the rat faeces, became infected with the eggs of the parasite which was then shed by the insect in larval form. In their turn the larvae were picked up by the rats in whose stomachs the adult nematodes developed. Fibiger examined sixty-one rats caught in one sugar refinery in Copenhagen. Forty of these animals had parasites and eggs in their stomachs and nine had cancers as well. The nature of the association between the parasites and the cancers remains a mystery to this day, for Fibiger's observations could not subsequently be confirmed.

CANCER PRODUCTION BY VIRUSES

Chicken leukosis, the first virus-induced cancer to be described, was investigated by Ellerman and Bang in 1908. Rous, as we have already mentioned, discovered his transmissible chick sarcoma in 1910–11. Twenty years later, Richard Shope (1932, 1933) published his descriptions of viruses which gave warts and skin cancers in rabbits. In 1936, Bittner found a non-cellular 'factor' involved in the genesis of breast cancers in some strains of mice. This is now called mammary tumour virus (MTV). Lucké (1938) observed that kidney carcinomas arising in the leopard frogs of Vermont could be transmitted to other frogs by cell-free filtrates. Thus, by the beginning of the Second World War there was substantial evidence that different viruses could induce cancers in several different species of animal. Some pathologists then, and one or two even now, rejected virus-induced tumours as true cancers and preferred to classify them as 'infectious granulomas' – but then the 'flat-earth' proponents are not even dejected (certainly not converted) by satellite-derived photographs – hence the truth of the old adage 'my mind is made up, do not confuse me with facts'.

After the war the pace of virus research accelerated, propelled by new techniques and instruments unknown before. Tissues were cultivated in incubators outside the body of the animal from which they derived and, like the animal's own cells, proved to be just as susceptible, not only to destruction by some viruses, but also to transformation into malignant cells. Cancers could thus be produced at will in an easily accessible way and the full fruits of such investigations have yet to be harvested.

Improvements in microscopy, and especially the use of electron microscopes with their greatly superior resolution and magnification, enabled the investigators not only to see virus particles in the cells of mouse and chicken cancers, but to see where they were produced in the cell and even to investigate the substructure of some of them, and the way in which they are assembled. New techniques in biochemistry – or molecular biology as it is now rechristened – especially with the use of radioactive 'tracers' allow the chemical stages in virus production to be followed in the cell and, as yet only potentially, the way in which the genetic material of the virus (DNA or RNA) is integrated with that of the cell, for it is in this integration that the secret of how viruses transform normal cells into malignant cells probably lies.

At this time, too, very young, immunologically immature animals began to be used to test the cancer-producing activity of new viruses (and, indeed, of chemicals as well).

VIRUS-INDUCED LEUKAEMIAS IN MICE

In 1951 Ludwik Gross described the production of leukaemia in C3H mice – with a very low spontaneous incidence of the disease – when the animals were injected, when one day old, with cell-free extracts from leukaemias arising in another strain of mice (AkR) with a high incidence of the disease. Leukaemias can be transmitted from mouse to mouse with very few cells, but Gross was cautious in using a filter which removed all cells, and so the leukaemias in the C3H mice can only have arisen by the action of a virus.

Leukaemias can also be induced in other strains of mice after irradiation, as Henry Kaplan has shown in a very elegant series of experiments and, once induced, these leukaemias are transmissible to other mice by cell-free (virus-containing) extracts. The implication here is clear. The mice irradiated by Kaplan must have carried a 'latent' leukaemia virus which was 'activated' by the radiation.

A second group of leukaemia-producing viruses for mice has been derived from other transplantable mouse tumours (not leukaemias). The virus isolated by Charlotte Friend in 1957 was obtained from the spleen of a Swiss strain mouse inoculated in infancy with a cell-free extract from Ehrlich's mouse carcinoma. At about the same time, Graffi and his colleagues in East Germany derived a different mouse leukaemia virus from a variety of transplantable mouse carcinomas and sarcomas. Other viruses have been turned up more recently but their provenance is identical – they were all associated with mice in a form in which they did not produce the disease but from whose tissues they could be isolated and increased in virulence.

POLYOMA VIRUS

When Ludwik Gross was describing the effect of his leukaemia virus on C3H mice he noticed that some of the mice had tumours of the parotid gland as well as leukaemia, and that whatever was producing these tumours was less sensitive to heat than the leukaemia virus. Sarah Stewart and her colleagues, in 1957, grew pieces of these tumours in tissue-culture with monkey-kidney cells (used normally to produce polio virus for vaccination). The cell-free fluids from these cultures, which were grown in an incubator at blood heat, were inoculated into newborn mice. The tumours which these mice developed included not only parotid gland sarcomas but also other primary tumours including those of the adrenal gland and the breast. Subsequently (1958), Bernice Eddy *et al.* found that hamsters developed tumours even more readily than mice with this virus – and so do rabbits, rats, guinea-pigs and even ferrets. This multiple action of this virus – which is quite unlike the mouse leukaemia viruses in its physical and chemical properties – led to its being called *poly*oma virus.

CELL TRANSFORMATION

One of the interesting properties of polyoma virus (which it shares with a number of others which contain DNA) is that, under certain conditions in tissue-culture *(in vitro)*, it *destroys* its host cells with the subsequent liberation of very large amounts of viruses, whereas in the animal *(in vivo)* it elicits tumours, i.e. it promotes the transformation of normal cells rather than their death.

This transformation can also be brought about in cells in culture and the way in which it occurs is the subject of much current research. The consensus of opinion would probably be that, in some way or other, the genetically-active portion of the virus – the DNA – becomes associated with, possibly actively part of, the cell's own DNA. One of the consequences of this interaction is malignancy for the cell as shown by the fact that, after transplantation into young animals of the same species as that from which the original cells were derived, tumours are produced. There is at least one other very important consequence of this transformation. The new race of cells – their daughters perpetuate the original properties – produce antigens which are absent from the original transformed cells and which are dependent for their formation upon the new genetic 'data' introduced by the virus. The new antigens are not components of the virus itself, which also has antigens distinct from those of the cell, and do not, in fact, appear to have a specific function, e.g. they are not new enzymes concerned with virus multiplication because the DNA-containing viruses do not, in general, multiply in the tumour cells which they induce.

The DNA-containing cancer-producing viruses form an interesting group. When polio viruses, for use in vaccines, began to be grown in cultures of monkey-kidney cells, much attention was paid to that normal kidney to see what monkey viruses were to be found in it. Obviously there was a danger that these would turn up in the final vaccine. One of those which did turn up was called simian virus 40 (SV40). This particular virus, which has now, of course, been excluded from the vaccines, appears to live in happy symbiosis with the cells of some species of monkey, but it is lethal for others and, more important, transforms normal cells of hamsters into tumour cells and will even transform human embryo cells in culture. Like polyoma virus, the DNA of SV40 is the infective material.

A cancer-producing virus from primates – even if it has only been shown to produce cancer in lower animals – takes us closer to the question of viruses and human cancer, but, since 1962, we have known that we can get closer still. In that year John Trentin and his colleagues in Houston, Texas, described the production of tumours in hamsters, inoculated when newborn with viruses of human origin, adenovirus 12 and 18. These adenoviruses – so-called because of their original isolation from human adenoidal tissue – only cause minor respiratory illnesses in man, such as sore throats and slight colds.

There are more than thirty different kinds of adenovirus of man, and monkey, chicken, cows and pigs have others, too; but not all of these produce cancer in hamsters and *none* has been implicated as a cause of cancer in man.

VIRUS HYBRIDIZATION

The SV40 virus, however, and some of the adenoviruses can take part in a fascinating hybridization which I have called the 'Trojan horse' phenomenon. Under certain conditions of co-cultivation the SV40 DNA can be wrapped up in the outer 'coat' of the adenovirus. The resulting hybrid is externally an adenovirus and in this guise can often gain access to cells which SV40 virus would be unable to penetrate. Inside the cell the cancer-producing SV40 DNA is liberated with dire consequences. It is not yet clear how widespread this phenomenon is, whether for example, the relatively harmless influenza virus can incorporate a piece of genetic material from a cancer-producing virus which it chances to encounter. Perhaps 'hybrid' influenza viruses have something to do with lung cancer in man – in association with cigarette-smoke, which undoubtedly plays the major role.

Other oncogenic viruses appear to be defective in different ways. Some of the Rous sarcoma viruses require a piece of genetic material from related viruses (which produce leukaemia in chickens) before they can be duplicated in the cell. A mouse sarcoma virus discovered by Jennifer Harvey at the London Hospital a year or two ago appears to be defective in a similar sense. It can multiply when the transformed cells divide, but is less able to convert cultured cells to malignancy unless a related mouse leukaemia virus is present.

These peculiarities of behaviour are fascinating by themselves and lead to much speculation about the origins of the oncogenic viruses. Some believe that most normal cells have within the genome a piece of 'malignant DNA' almost like an unfused bomb. Along comes an X-ray, a chemical carcinogen or a complementary piece of DNA or RNA from a virus, and the fuse is lit.

VIRUSES AND THE EPIDEMIOLOGY OF HUMAN CANCER

The hypothesis that leukaemia in man could be linked to viruses, or virus-like organisms, must be flexible enough to accommodate the possibility of 'inheritance' in the sense in which mouse RNA tumour viruses are inherited, and the further probability that, whereas the virus may be responsible for the conversion of normal cell to malignant cell, the *disease* itself may be elicited by other factors, for example chemical or physical carcinogens.

Researches are now being vigorously conducted into the epidemiology of leukaemia in man. Many reports have appeared of 'outbreaks' of the disease in children which have occurred within small areas and over short periods of time. These have been accepted by some as evidence for an epidemic – like spread of the disease. *What* might be spreading has not, however, been discussed. If it is a cancer-producing virus, then it is probably less like the mouse or avian RNA-containing leukaemia viruses which are spread vertically, from mother to offspring, and more like the DNA-containing viruses such as polyoma, SV40 and the adenoviruses which spread horizontally.

Again, the 'trigger' for the disease may be a virus, such as measles, which spreads horizontally, but which is not regarded, conventionally, as a cancer-producing virus. There is some evidence from one of the reports on clustering which centred round a school in Niles, Illinois, in the USA, that an unidentified virus was circulating in the child community, and producing a rheumatic disease.

There are further difficulties in such studies : first 'clusters of reporting' have to be differentiated from true case-clusters; second, aggregation of cases must occur by chance alone; and, third, the time of clinical diagnosis may be variably related to the time of onset of the disease.

The leukaemic tissues in mouse and fowl harbour the causative virus which may not only be visualized in the cells by electron microscopy but may also be concentrated by centrifugation and studied virologically. The analogous situation does not appear to occur in man. Some investigators claim to have seen virus-like particles in cells or plasma from leukaemic individuals; others have seen mycoplasmas (PPLO) and G. Negroni, of the Imperial Cancer Research Fund, has isolated such a mycoplasma from the bone-marrow of leukaemic individuals. This organism has a filterable phase (in which it behaves like a virus) and leukaemic patients have neutralizing antibodies to it in their sera.

Epidemiologists must take account both of the virologists' findings in animal cancer and the mode of transmission of mouse and fowl leukaemia viruses, when they design their investigations. They should certainly not assume that a specific *oncogenic* agent is being propagated in a 'case-cluster' but should, if possible, survey for any and all transmissible pathogens – for any, or all, of these could be the appropriate trigger.

One must now admit that the search for an aetiological agent for the other form of cancer (the Burkitt lymphoma of children in Africa) which appears to show an 'epidemicity' has, until recently, also been pursued along conventional lines.

Since the days of the first English medical missionaries in Uganda, there have been records of African children with rapidly-growing malignant tumours in the jaws. Denis Burkitt first noticed in 1958 that the tumours in the jaws were sometimes accompanied by tumours in the kidneys, adrenals, liver, salivary glands and ovaries. With the recognition of a clinical entity came now the histological identification of the tumour, by J. N. P. Davies, as a lymphoma. In the next few years, Burkitt pursued the age and geographical distribution of the disease throughout Africa. It was soon apparent that the tumours were not found in Ugandan children less than two years old, and that few cases were seen in adults. The peak age distribution was between six and nine years (29–34 per cent). However, in an emigrant 'susceptible' population from Rwanda and Burundi 26 per cent of the cases occurred in those older than thirty-three. Furthermore, the geographical distribution in terms of height, temperature and rainfall was found to parallel very closely that for insect vectors of disease such as yellow-fever and malaria. The hunt was then begun for a specific virus which, from its flying 'syringe',

79

could transmit the disease. The virus reservoir could, of course, equally well be animal as human because some of the insect virus vectors are not species-specific.

A number of different viruses has been found in association with Burkitt tumour tissue, either by electron microscopy or by direct isolation, or both. These include vaccinia, herpes simplex, reovirus 3 and a herpes-like virus which was first seen by Epstein and Barr, and is thus known as EB virus. In addition, Dalldorf and Bergamini found some mycoplasmas from cases in Nairobi. Vaccinia, herpes simplex and the mycoplasmas are currently considered to be 'passengers' rather than 'drivers' and interest now centres on reovirus 3 and EB virus.

It was reasonable to suppose that the Burkitt tumour might be found in other areas of the world with geographical parameters similar to those of central Africa. Indeed cases have been described from New Guinea and Brazil. However, there can now be no doubt that *true* Burkitt lymphomas do occur outside these tropical areas and epidemiologists are required to take a closer look at the precise implications of the original insect-borne virus hypothesis.

The EB virus was first noticed in some cells of a continuous culture of lymphoblast-like cells derived from a Burkitt tumour. It is now clear that most of the American or New Guinea Burkitt lymphomas which can be grown as cell-lines also harbour this virus. In addition it has been seen in non-Burkitt lymphoma cell lines and in lines originating from lymphoid cells of apparently normal individuals in the USA. The most intriguing finding, however, has been that of Henle, Henle and Diehl of Philadelphia. The EB virus was seen to be associated with infectious mono-nucleosis (glandular fever) and the association was confirmed by serological studies. We have, then, a virus, apparently trans-missible by cell-to-cell contact – like other herpesviruses – and found in association with lymphoblastic cells of cell lines from Burkitt tumours, lymphomas, infectious mononucleosis, and normal lymphoid tissues of man. It is scarcely surprising that the sera of a high percentage of American children and adults, as well as Burkitt tumour patients, react positively with complement-fixing antigens from these cell lines.

Reovirus 3, another candidate virus, has a widespread distribution in man and animals where its normal mode of spread is faecal-oral. Mosquito transmission between mice has been claimed by Parker *et al.* in Australia, and there are recent data from Stanley's laboratory in Perth on the induction of *mouse* lymphomas by this virus.

The exact significance of either EB virus or reovirus 3 in the aetiology of the Burkitt lymphoma remains to be determined, for it must be admitted that there is no direct evidence to show how either virus could be transmitted and no human or animal reservoir has yet been detected. There are, of course, other possibilities than that of direct spread and these might have more relevance to those cases which have occurred outside the tropical areas of Africa, New Guinea and Brazil. The first is that the Burkitt tumour might replace childhood leukaemias in these areas and there have been suggestions of a deficit in these in Africa compared with Europe and the USA. New data from Mulago Hospital, however, indicate that childhood leukaemia in Ugandan children may hitherto have been missed. The second possibility follows the line of thought already developed for leukaemia, i.e. that either reovirus 3 or EB virus may initiate the fundamental cell changes, but that the 'triggers' for the development of the disease may, in tropical countries, be insect-borne viruses or parasites (such as malaria). In this way the epidemiology of the disease in these areas would still be meaningful.

There is evidence that Burkitt tumour cells carry antigens against which the patient himself may be able to produce antibodies. Immune rejection is thought to play a part in successful chemotherapy of the disease which, rarely, regresses spontaneously. If clinically-apparent tumours have been observed to regress this is just the tip of the iceberg and *many* clinically-inapparent tumours, under African conditions, will have been extinguished in this way. Tumours may progress, therefore, in individuals incapacitated immunologically by insect-borne disease in Africa, etc., but in other ways, and more rarely, in other parts of the world.

It is reasonable to believe, at this time, that EB virus, in particular, plays a role in the abnormal multiplication of lymphoid cells. Its wide distribution and horizontal spread (in infectious mononucleosis) may have implications for tumours of lymphoid origin, but the epidemiology of leukaemia, or the Burkitt lymphoma may not be comprehensible in terms of the distribution of a single virus, and we shall undoubtedly have to take into consideration more of the environment of the leukaemic individual, whether this be pre- or post-natal, internal or external, chemical or physical.

Dr Robert Baldwin will be discussing how carcinogens act and the immunological consequences of the neo-antigens induced by both carcinogens and viruses in the next section, and I shall help to set the scene for him by describing briefly the historical sequence of ideas about the biochemical differences between normal cells and their malignant counterparts.

THE BIOCHEMISTRY OF TUMOURS

The first, and by all accounts the most popular, theory was that which Otto Warburg enunciated in 1931 in his book *The Metabolism of Tumours*. Warburg had noticed changes in the glycolytic and respiratory enzyme systems in tumour cells, which differentiated them from normal cells (or, at least, from most normal cells), and he regarded these, and their induction, as the key changes. Farber (1968) has pointed out, however, that Warburg had, perforce, studied a wide variety of primary tumours and most of these were in an advanced state biologically – in a late stage of progression, as Leslie Foulds would have described them.

Then came, as we have already seen, efficient methods of transplanting animal tumours. In this way larger amounts of more homogeneous material became available and Warburg's original generalization appeared to be less tenable. No single change or sequence of biochemical changes could at first be correlated with malignancy, although there were quantitative differences in the concentration of different components. More intensive investigation, however, showed that some tumours had lost enzymes or proteins in comparison with their normal counterparts and, as we have already seen, some appeared to have gained new antigens of, as yet, undetermined function.

Cancers are not uniform in their properties, and Morris and others have studied with great intensity the biochemistry of a series of rat liver cancers which they have called 'minimum deviation hepatomas'. In Foulds' terminology these appear to be much less 'advanced' than any others which have been studied in a comparable way, and they closely resemble normal liver in their biochemical properties.

It may not be reasonable even to attempt to compare the mechanism of induction of cancer by viruses, chemicals or radiation, but the only satisfactory generalization at present— which fits equally the clinical data from man and the experimental data from animals—is that the change which cells undergo from normal to malignant is not a single event but a multi-sequence process in which cells or even tissues gradually begin to show the biological properties which characterize malignancy, and which have been discussed in Dr Lajtha's chapter in this book. The time-scale on which these progressive events occur may be far from uniform and, whereas a virus may bring about a complete transformation in a few hours, chemicals, hormones and radiation may take months or years.

CHAPTER IV

THE PRESENT DIRECTION OF CANCER RESEARCH

R. W. BALDWIN

CHEMICAL INDUCTION OF CANCER

There are two reasons for studying cancer-producing agents (carcinogens), whether chemical, physical or viral. First, a knowledge of the nature of carcinogens is an essential part of modern biological technology required to ensure that such substances are not unwittingly introduced into our environment. As we shall see, the concept of cancer prevention has played an important role over the last fifty years or more in leading to the identification of chemical substances causing cancer, particularly those types which occur more frequently in certain industrial workers than in the general population. The notion of cancer prevention is of much greater importance at the present time with regard to the problems of lung cancer, since it is clear that the disease would be largely prevented if cigarette smoking was to cease.

Second, progress in understanding the mechanisms of cancer induction (carcinogenesis), whereby a normal cell is transformed into a cancer cell, has also developed from fundamental studies on the chemistry of cancer-inducing agents. The initial belief that only a few substances with highly specific properties would have the capacity to induce cancer has not been realized. On the contrary, the outstanding feature of carcinogenesis is the immense diversity of active substances. Only relatively recently has it been possible to discern any common pattern of behaviour for the many carcinogens in their reactions within cells. It now seems that whilst various carcinogens initially operate by different biochemical pathways, they may produce similar, or in some cases identical, changes of key factors associated with the hereditary properties of the cell.

CANCER AND THE ENVIRONMENT

Oil and Skin Cancer

Dr Harris has already described the pioneer studies of Kennaway and the Royal Cancer Hospital group which lead to the discovery of the polycyclic hydrocarbon carcinogens.

Historically, cancer of the skin arising from contact with oils was a major factor leading to the identification of pure chemical substances with carcinogenic properties. Cancer of the skin in the Lancashire cotton industry was recognized as an industrial hazard and became notifiable in 1920 as an industrial disease. Later, in 1953, specifications were included in the Mule Spinning (Health) Special Regulations defining the nature of the oils which may be used in this process. These regulations together with changes in industrial techniques then reduced the incidence of skin cancer in the cotton industry, but the risk was not completely removed. Despite this historical precedent and the knowledge that certain mineral oils contain carcinogenic substances, there are still reports of skin cancer in industrial workers. This is a particular problem in the engineering and metallurgical industries as a result of exposure of tool-setters to cutting oils used to lubricate and cool machines. It has been estimated, for example, that one in every 1,000 toolsetters contracts cancer of the scrotum in the Birmingham area. This was the subject of considerable press publicity recently following the court award of £10,000 to the widow of a Walsall toolsetter who died from scrotal cancer. He had worked for fourteen years as a toolsetter and his job involved leaning over machines which brought his body in contact with oil. The obvious answer to this problem is to ensure that only safe oils are used. These would be more costly to produce and so, without statutory regulations such as those governing oils used in the cotton industry, it is unlikely that such a measure could be rapidly and totally introduced. The answer at the present time, therefore, would seem to be an insistence on a much higher standard of hygiene, avoidance of contact with oils, and periodic medical examination of workers where oils are extensively used. Above all, it is necessary to educate workers about the potential risk of oil exposure and for thus purpose HM Factory Inspectors have produced a series of cautionary notices.

With the ever increasing use of oils and oil products in modern technological processes, there is a need for a much more effective communication between industry and oil producers, the medical researcher and government departments concerned with industrial health. The objective of the medical scientist is to identify potential health risks; he has no desire to see his experimental findings confirmed some time later by epidemiological studies on industrial workers.

Aromatic Amines and Bladder Cancer

The early history of the association of aromatic amines and bladder cancer has already been recounted (pp. 69–70).

The manufacture of 2-naphthylamine in the British dyestuffs industry was largely abandoned by 1950, and completely so by 1952. Benzidine continued to be produced for much longer under a 'Code of Working Practice' but in June 1965, immediately after a case of bladder cancer had been diagnosed in a worker, this plant of 'advanced protective design' was closed and production stopped. Subsequently the only British plant for the production of 1-naphthylamine was closed in December 1965 when bladder cancer was diagnosed in one of the twenty-five employees. Hence, by the end of 1965, manufacture of aromatic amines known to cause bladder cancer had ceased in this country.

Whilst the nature of the hazard of industrial exposure to aromatic amines was recognized and eventually acted upon in the industries concerned in their manufacture, other users in this country, notably some sections of the rubber industry, were much slower to respond. For instance, naphthylamines were introduced in the late 1920s into the chemical manufacture of antioxidants used in the production of rubber and cables. The scattered nature of the rubber industry made it more difficult to survey the workers but, by 1954, evidence was published showing that there was an occupational risk of rubber workers dying from bladder cancer. Following this, the Rubber Manufacturers Employers Association (RMEA) set up a Health Unit in 1957 to provide diagnostic facilities for their workers and in 1961 issued an explanatory booklet *(Papilloma of the Bladder in the Rubber Industry)*. The large rubber manufacturers being members of RMEA were aware of the bladder cancer hazard, but many of the smaller manufacturers were not. Hence carcinogenic aromatic amines

86

have continued to be imported, since British manufacture ceased around 1950, and used in some sections of the cable-making industry at least up to 1964, and this occasioned some public comment following the report in 1965 of an inquest on a former cable worker who died of inoperable bladder cancer many years after exposure to 2-naphthylamine. Legislative control, embodied in the Carcinogenic Substances Regulations and Carcinogenic Substances (Prohibition of Importation) Order, came into effect by December 1967. These regulations ban the import or use, except under licence by the Chief Inspector of Factories, of a number of substances including 2-naphthylamine, benzidine and 4-aminodiphenyl so that at last the hazard of exposure to these compounds is under control. Nevertheless, it is a long time since the discovery of bladder cancer among German aniline workers in 1895 and one wonders how many workers died of bladder cancer because of the lack of effective communication between government, industry and the medical profession.

CHEMISTRY OF CANCER INDUCTION

Following the discovery of the major classes of cancer-inducing chemicals such as polycyclic hydrocarbons, aromatic amines, aminoazo dyes and nitroso compounds, literally hundreds of different chemicals have been tested with the aim of defining as precisely as possible the chemical properties responsible for carcinogenic action. It is now widely accepted that this approach has not provided any clear-cut criteria by which carcinogenic potency can be defined in simple chemical terms. Undoubtedly, this is because, in most cases, cancer-inducing chemicals undergo a most complex series of changes in the body as a result of metabolism. In contemporary research, therefore, much more attention is being paid to identifying the various metabolites (products of metabolism) both with respect to their carcinogenic properties and chemical composition. By this means, it is hoped to elucidate the initial steps in the carcinogenic process. This type of research only became possible in recent years with the development of very sensitive methods for locating breakdown products of carcinogens in the body. Foremost amongst these methods has been the use of chemical carcinogens in which one or more of the constituent atoms are radioactive. For example, carcinogens can be synthesized in which either the carbon or hydrogen atoms are radioactive. These radioactive atoms emit radiations which can be detected and quantitated using specialized recording instruments such as Geiger-Müller counters or, better still, scintillation counters. In the scintillation counter, each radioactive particle or ray emitted by the atom produces a minute flash of light in a specially prepared crystal and this light in turn is detected by a type of electric eye. Using these 'tracer' techniques it is possible, for example, to administer very small amounts of a carcinogen to an animal and follow the fate of the substance as it is distributed to various tissues in the body. The rate of metabolism can also be determined by measuring the amount of radioactivity excreted and it is then possible to use the radioactivity as a marker in chemical studies on the isolation and identification of the excreted metabolites.

It is difficult to summarize these highly technical studies in simple terms, but some idea of the general approaches and achievements can be given by reference to two examples.

Aromatic Amines

As already described, aromatic amines constitute an important class of chemical carcinogens since many of these substances have proved to be potentially hazardous to man. One compound 2-acetylaminofluorene (AAF; Figure 18), initially investigated because of its insecticidal properties, was found to be highly carcinogenic and is now used extensively for experimental cancer studies. This chemical is highly carcinogenic when fed to rats, producing cancer at a number of sites but particularly in liver and breast tissues. The observation that cancer was generally produced in tissues distant from the site of oral entry, whereas no cancers generally arose in skin following repeated application, pointed to the possibility that metabolic breakdown products may be the active cancer-producing agents. In order to test this hypothesis, extensive studies were carried out to identify the various metabolities and this work indicated that many were formed by a process of 'hydroxylation'. Essentially this involves substitution of hydrogen atoms by hydroxyl (OH) groups (Figure 18) and this process is a major route by which the body prepares foreign substances, such as drugs, for excretion by making them soluble in water. When, however, the various metabolites were

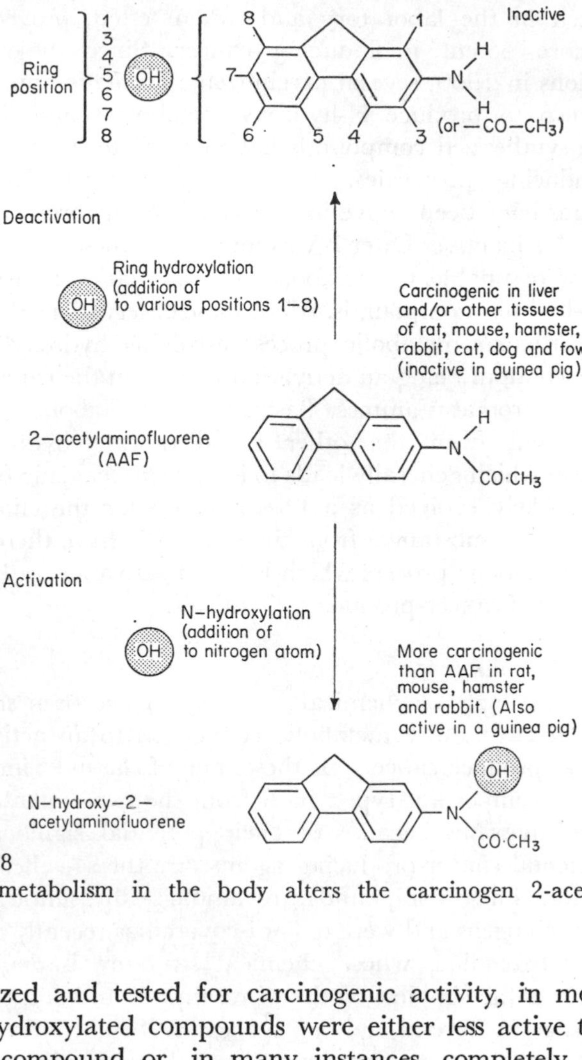

FIGURE 18

How metabolism in the body alters the carcinogen 2-acetylamino-fluorene.

synthesized and tested for carcinogenic activity, in most cases these hydroxylated compounds were either less active than the parent compound or, in many instances, completely inactive. Such observations are compatible with the view that hydroxylation of chemical carcinogens, like drugs, represents a process designed to inactivate and prepare for excretion. It was then discovered that an unexpected metabolite of the carcinogen was also excreted in the urine and in this case the hydroxyl substituent was on the nitrogen atom, rather than on one of the carbon atoms (Figure 18). This so-called N-hydroxy compound was later

89

synthesized in the laboratory and, when tested, proved to be much more potent in inducing cancer. Since these crucial observations in 1960, several carcinogenic aromatic amines have been shown to produce N-hydroxy metabolites and, in every case, the synthesized compounds have proved to have enhanced cancer-inducing properties. Also, in some cases, N-hydroxy compounds have been active in species where the original parent compound is inactive. Later it was found that these unsusceptible animals were unable to metabolise the aromatic amines to the active N-hydroxy compounds. All of these observations thus point to this particular metabolic process involving hydroxylation of the nitrogen atom being an activation process in the carcinogenic response to aromatic amines. Basically this metabolic process is little different from the other so-called ring hydroxylation metabolism which generally leads to loss of carcinogenic function, and most likely evolved as a host reaction for the elimination of foreign toxic substances from the body. We have therefore an aberrant metabolic process which leads to activation rather than deactivation of cancer-producing chemicals.

Nitroso Compounds
Several other types of chemical carcinogen have been shown in recent years to require metabolic conversion to an active form in order to produce cancer. Of these, one of the most interesting and perhaps important types, both from the experimental viewpoint and possibly because of their potential significance as environmental cancer-producing agents, are the so-called nitroso compounds. These compounds are amongst the simplest of all known carcinogens and were only discovered as recently as 1956. Dimethylnitrosamine, whose chemical structure is depicted in Figure 19, is the simplest of the nitrosamines and is a powerful liver poison in several animal species. When, however, it is administered to rats at a very low dose so that acute liver damage is minimized, the animals eventually develop cancer of the liver and kidney. Significantly, also, it is possible to induce cancer following only a single dose of the chemical. The cancer so induced may not become apparent until many months after this single exposure although it is known that the dimethylnitrosamine is rapidly metabolised and may persist for only a matter of hours.

Another important feature of the nitrosamines is their wide

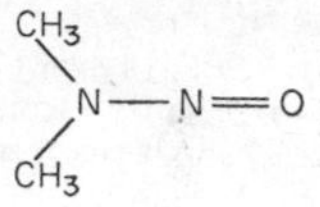

Dimethylnitrosamine
(other nitroso compounds can be formed
by replacing the two-armed CH_3 groups)

FIGURE 19
Carcinogenic nitroso compounds.

range of action which is probably greater than that of any other type of carcinogen. Although the rat has been mostly used in experimental studies, various nitrosamines obtained by varying the chemical nature of the side chains (Figure 19) are carcinogenic in a range of species including monkeys and other mammals, as well as birds and fish. Moreover nitrosamines produce cancer in many organs including kidney, lung, oesophagus, bladder, and even brain.

As already indicated, nitroso compounds are very rapidly metabolised in the body and it is believed that they are not in themselves carcinogenic but that this is a property of some metabolic breakdown product. The nature of the intermediate biologically active metabolites has not been firmly established, but a probable sequence of reactions for dimethylnitrosamine has been formulated (Figure 20). From these studies it appears that the essential metabolic step in the degradation of the chemical may be the formation of an intermediate product ($*CH_2$) which, because of its extreme instability, is only short lived. Such a highly reactive metabolite will however, be capable of modifying cellular constituents and thus produce permanent damage in the cell which eventually may lead to cancer formation.

This brief outline of current ideas regarding the mechanism of action of chemical carcinogens has of necessity had to be simple since many of the concepts involve sophisticated chemical ideas. An important feature, well illustrated in the two examples, has been the shift in emphasis towards the study of carcinogen metabolism, and from this the concept of the so-called reactive carcinogenic intermediates has evolved. This has meant a move away from the conventional chemical approach towards the use of newer biochemical methods, particularly those designed for identifying extremely small amounts of metabolites many of

91

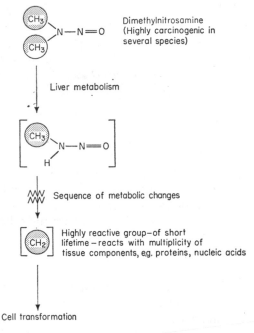

FIGURE 20

Probable metabolism of dimethylnitrosamine leading to reactive metabolites.

which are highly unstable and therefore difficult to isolate. The concept of reactive carcinogenic metabolites is now being explored in almost all classes of chemical carcinogens, and the hope is that this type of approach in defining the nature of the reactive carcinogen metabolites will also make possible the characterization of the *cell* component involved in the interaction.

MOLECULAR BIOLOGY OF CANCER INDUCTION

The cellular and molecular mechanisms of cancer induction by chemical carcinogens are still largely unknown, but this is hardly surprising since the many intricate processes involved in normal cell function are only partially understood. It is generally accepted that the transformation of a normal cell to a cancer cell is irreversible, leading to the development of cells with new growth properties and which fail to respond to the controlling mechanisms of the body. Because of this, it is highly likely that this transformation involves changes in the hereditary apparatus of the cell responsible for normal cell development and replication. This, as already discussed in Chapter I, is located in the nucleus of the cell in the twin-stranded chainlike molecules of deoxyribonucleic acid (DNA) grouped into chromosomes. These DNA molecules have a long backbone made up of repeating groups of phosphate and a five-carbon sugar (deoxyribose) with side groups called bases at regular intervals. It is the arrangement of these four bases guanine, adenine, cytosine and thymine, which act as a template providing, in coded form, specifications for the synthesis of the many thousands of proteins required by the cell.

Two general mechanisms have been proposed to account for cell transformation by chemical carcinogens. The first holds that the essential mechanism involves direct interaction of the reactive carcinogen metabolite with DNA, thereby inducing chemical modification of the DNA. The second hypothesis proposes that the primary targets for carcinogen-interaction are cytoplasmic proteins. Although it is not yet clear how these latter changes may cause the cell to acquire new permanent heritable characteristics, many feel that this hypothesis best fits the observed facts.

Carcinogen-DNA Interaction

It has been known since 1940 that heritable changes can be induced in micro-organisms or flies by exposure to chemicals,

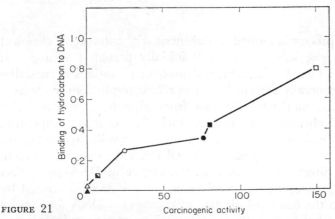

FIGURE 21

Showing the correlation of the extent of binding to mouse-skin DNA of a series of hydrocarbons of varying carcinogenic activity.

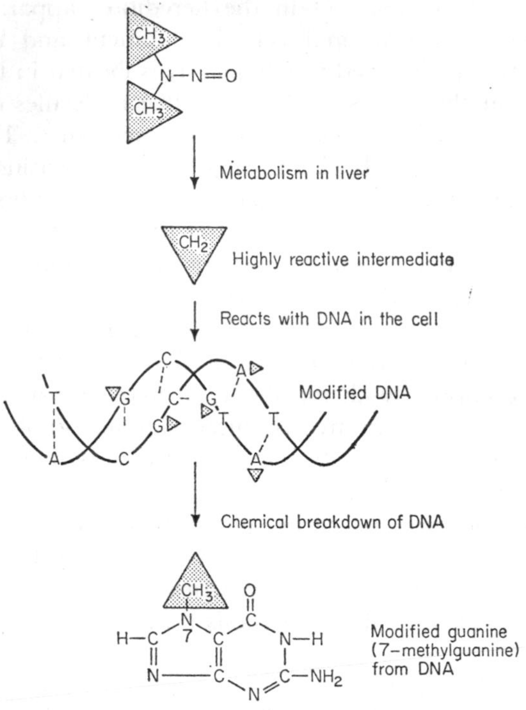

FIGURE 22
Modification of deoxyribonucleic acid by metabolites of the carcinogen dimethylnitrosamine.

and this process is termed mutagenesis. For instance, a chemical (mustard gas, sulphur mustard) initially prepared as a poison gas in the First World War, will produce mutations in fruit flies and it is generally agreed that these effects result from interaction with DNA. Similarly examples from almost all of the major classes of chemical carcinogens, including nitroso compounds, aromatic amines, aminoazo dyes and polycyclic hydrocarbons, have been found to interact with cell DNA. In many cases there is also a direct correlation with the degree of DNA-interaction and the potency of the carcinogen. This is well illustrated by studies on the extent of binding to mouse skin DNA for a series of polycyclic hydrocarbons of varying carcinogenic potency (Figure 21).

94

In a few examples, the chemical nature of the DNA modification has been defined in fairly precise terms. For instance, nitroso compounds, which probably produce a highly reactive metabolite, react with cell DNA and, when the modified DNA was broken down by chemical methods, two of the bases, guanine and to a lesser extent adenine, were found to be altered. Thus treatment of rats with dimethylnitrosamine resulted in the formation of a modified DNA in liver and kidney in which the normal guanine component was converted to 7-methylguanine (Figure 22).

Studies with other carcinogens, because of their greater chemical complexity, are not yet as advanced. In many instances, however, progress is being made in defining the extent of the interaction with tissue DNA in relation to the carcinogenic activity of the chemicals. From such quantitative studies it is hoped that some clear-cut relationship will be produced showing that DNA-reaction is a critical process in carcinogenesis. At the

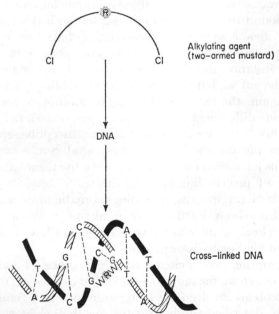

FIGURE 23
Cross-linking between the guanine bases of the two polynucleotide chains of DNA by an alkylating agent.

same time, efforts are being made to understand how modifications to nucleic acids may lead to the conversion of normal cells to cancer cells. For instance the action of so-called alkylating agents like sulphur mustard is thought to be due to cross-linking of the two strands of the DNA molecule (Figure 23). In other cases where the effect of carcinogen interaction with DNA may not produce such profound changes, the situation is not yet understood. It may be, for instance, that the outcome of treatment with a carcinogen will depend upon the balance between the degree of modification of DNA caused by the carcinogen and the efficiency of the cell in repairing or tolerating DNA damage.

Carcinogen-Protein Interaction

Not all cancer biochemists accept that binding of carcinogens to DNA is the critical cell interaction leading to cancer, since similar but much greater carcinogen-protein binding may occur. The first demonstration of such interactions, reported in 1947, showed that a carcinogenic aminoazo dye (4-dimethylaminoazobenzene) became bound to liver proteins of rats fed with this dye (Figure 24). Since then, a wide range of correlations have been established between protein binding and carcinogenic activity of aminoazo dyes. For instance, these carcinogens are only active towards the liver in the rat and this is the tissue in which protein binding occurs. Again, the extent of binding of aminoazo dyes to liver proteins in different species appears to be related to their susceptibility to these carcinogens and unsusceptible species like the guinea pig do not form protein-bound complexes. Similar correlations have been established between the tissue- and species-specificity of protein binding and the carcinogenicity of many other types of carcinogens, including aromatic amines and polycyclic hydrocarbons. Furthermore, in almost every case, inactive chemicals closely similar to known carcinogens have not had this property of binding to tissue proteins.

In attempting to elucidate the significance of carcinogen-protein interaction, the nature of the bound carcinogen metabolite and the proteins involved are being examined in several systems. As already described, studies on the metabolism of carcinogens have indicated that many undergo a process of metabolic activation. These findings in turn are now making possible predictions

96

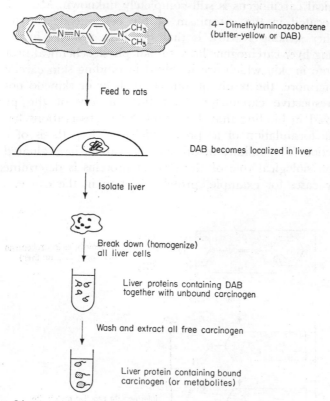

FIGURE 24
Binding of liver carcinogen, 4-dimethylaminoazobenzene, to liver proteins.

about the mechanism of carcinogen-interaction with protein (or nucleic acids). For instance, Figure 25 illustrates a possible sequence of events leading to the formation of protein-bound metabolites of an aminoazo dye. This involves conversion of the carcinogen to a reactive N-hydroxy metabolite (unstable) which then reacts with sulphur-containing amino acids of the proteins. Many of the details of these reactions have still to be worked out, but the essential feature is that the metabolic changes which make a carcinogen more active can be implicated in the process of carcinogen-protein binding.

The function of the proteins involved in the binding with

97

chemical carcinogens is still completely unknown. Most of these are located in the cytoplasm of the cell outside the nucleus. Another striking feature is that the liver proteins involved in binding liver carcinogens have similar physicochemical properties to those in skin which are involved in binding skin carcinogens. Furthermore, the resultant cancers of liver or skin do not bind the respective carcinogens and little if any of the proteins involved in binding may be found. Such observations have led to the formulation of a 'protein deletion' hypothesis of cancer induction. The validity of this concept cannot be evaluated until the physiological role of the deleted proteins is determined. In many cases for example, protein deletion in the cancer cell is

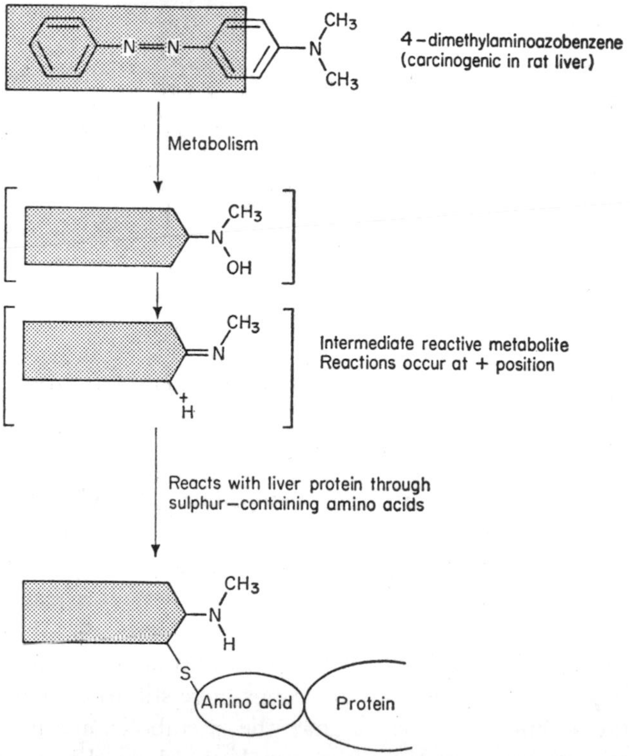

FIGURE 25

Possible sequence of metabolic changes leading to the binding of a metabolite of the carcinogen 4-dimethylaminoazobenzene to liver protein.

accompanied by an increased growth potential suggesting that these proteins may be involved in growth control.

This wealth of evidence on the binding of carcinogens to proteins and their subsequent deletion from cancer cells makes it difficult to exclude the possibility that these reactions are important in carcinogenesis. It is difficult, however, to postulate how such reactions involving cytoplasmic proteins could lead to the genetic change which is the characteristic feature of the cancer cell. One explanation to overcome these difficulties has been derived from work on the control of enzyme synthesis and activity in micro-organisms. This suggests that carcinogens interact with proteins which act as repressors controlling the function of genes. Deletion or inactivation of the repressor proteins by carcinogens may produce a series of changes which result in the release or unmasking of genes that are suppressed in the normal cell and, by this means, the cell acquires new characteristics.

At present, there is insufficient evidence to decide whether DNA or protein is the primary cellular site for modification by carcinogens, and sponsors of the rival theories will continue to work in support of their cause. As a result of these efforts, it may ultimately be found that both points of view have to be accommodated, since it is not impossible that the carcinogenic process may result from a number of different, biomolecular pathways related in some complex fashion to reaction of metabolites with both DNA and protein.

IMMUNITY AND CANCER

Immunological systems in mammals, whether man or mouse, are now generally recognized as playing a much more fundamental role than simply providing protection against infectious diseases. This changing view of the role of immunology has stemmed largely from studies on the mechanisms of tissue graft rejection. Cross-grafts of skin between adult mice of two different strains are normally rejected, since the recipient mouse recognizes markers (antigens) on the skin graft as foreign, and this evokes an immunological response comparable to the body's reaction to other foreign material such as bacteria and viruses (Figure 26). In man, the problem of immunological rejection of grafts has been dramatically highlighted by the death of several heart

99

transplant patients even though they had survived the operative procedure.

Returning to the mouse, experimenters found that whilst skin grafts were rejected in normal adult animals, this was not so if foetal or new-born mice were injected with cells from the donor

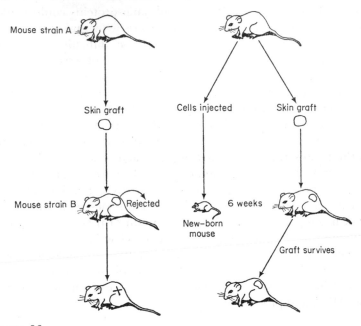

FIGURE 26

Induction of immunological tolerance.

Induction of specific immunological tolerance to grafted skin in mice. Skin grafts between adult mice of two strains A and B are rejected because the skin contains markers (antigens) different from those of the recipient. Injecting cells from A-strain mice into new-born B-strain mice renders B-strain mice tolerant to the antigens. In adult mice, skin now can be grafted.

mouse strain (Figure 26). Under these circumstances, the treated mice, when they became adult, accepted skin grafts from the mouse strain whose cells were injected at birth. That is, the mice were rendered 'immunologically tolerant' to the tissue antigens in the skin graft. These observations led to the formulation of the concept of 'self' and 'non-self', the idea being that the immuno-

100

logical system which 'matures' at birth or soon after is essentially a surveillance system evolved to protect the body from foreign cells of all sorts. Under these conditions the term 'foreign' means cells or other antigenic substances, which the host's immunological system does not come into contact with or 'see' during the early stages of development. In the skin grafting example (Figure 26) the mice injected at birth with cells from another strain accepted these foreign cells as 'self' and thus became 'tolerant' to skin grafts from this strain. This concept of immunological self-recognition has proved to have far-reaching consequences and led to the award of the Nobel Prize for Medicine in 1960 to Sir Peter Medawar, now Director of the National Institute for Medical Research, and Sir Macfarlane Burnet who was then Director of the Walter and Eliza Hall Institute of Medical Research in Melbourne, Australia.

The immunological self-recognition hypothesis implies that cells which gain new antigens at some stage after the recognition phase in the host, usually ending a few days after birth, will be identified as foreign and as such should be open to immunological attack. Therefore, if in the transformation of normal cells to cancer cells by treatment with chemical carcinogens, or viruses, new, cancer-specific antigens are produced, the cancer cells should be recognized as foreign by the body. Contemporary research in cancer immunology is concerned with establishing whether cancers of different aetiologies possess these specific cancer antigens and how effective they are in provoking cancer rejection in the host. Such studies, it is hoped, may lead to the development of new methods for cancer treatment.

IMMUNOLOGICAL TREATMENT OF CANCER

The idea of curing cancer by some form of immunological treatment is not particularly new; one of the earliest studies was made in 1903 by Paul Ehrlich, the pioneer of immunology and chemotherapy. In these early studies, remarkable 'cures' of animal cancers were frequently observed, but it is now recognized that much of this work is completely valueless because of inadequate experimental methods. Hence, in most investigations, the cancers which were cured had been transplanted into normal animals and these were, therefore, rejected in the same way as skin is rejected. These many investigations, carried out against a background of almost total ignorance of the science of transplantation immunology, produced an atmosphere of complete chaos and the early hopes that vaccination would lead to a cure for cancer were replaced by a total condemnation of this approach.

A more scientific approach to the problem of immunological treatment of cancer only became possible around the 1950s, following the elucidation of the basic rules of tissue transplantation and the development of inbred strains of animals. Inbred strains are produced by the laborious, and time-consuming, procedure of brother-to-sister mating for a minimum of twenty consecutive generations, and the animals can then be considered as replicas of each other just as are a pair of identical human twins. In genetic terms, animals of a particular strain are isologous (syngeneic), carrying identical sets of genes. This means that individual animals each possess the same complement of transplantation (histocompatibility) antigens so that, as in identical twins, it is possible to transplant skin between them.

CANCER–SPECIFIC ANTIGENS

Once these inbred strains of animals became available, it was possible to investigate whether experimentally-induced cancers acquired new antigens which were not present in normal tissues. In order to do this, normal animals were exposed to grafts of induced cancers in such a manner that the cancer cells were not able to grow unchecked, but which allowed the host to produce an immunological reaction against the presumptive cancer antigens. This can be achieved as illustrated in Figure 27 by implanting cancer cells which have been rendered incapable of continuous growth by exposure to a large dose of X-rays. Usually the treatment with irradiated cancer cells is repeated several times to increase the degree of resistance. When animals treated in this fashion are then inoculated with living cancer cells of the same cancer line, they are, in many cases, capable of rejecting the cancer graft, although this grows in control animals treated with irradiated *normal* tissues. Cancer cells inactivated in other ways such as treatment with cancer chemotherapeutic drugs may also be used for this purpose. More vigorous methods, such as

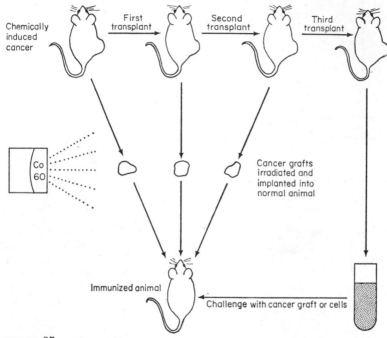

FIGURE 27

Showing how immunity can be produced against chemically-induced cancer in normal rats by implantation of radiation-killed cancer cells.

heating, inactivate both cancer cell and antigens so that cells treated in this manner will not produce resistance.

Another more simple method by which cancer immunity can be evoked is to implant viable grafts of the cancer, allow these to develop for a number of days and then surgically excise the developing growth (Figure 28). Again animals treated in this manner will reject a further implant of the same cancer.

Over the past decade, these methods have been applied in studies of the immunology of a variety of experimentally induced cancers, and in most, but not all, it has been possible to produce varying degrees of immunity. The situation is not as simple as that observed in resistance to infectious diseases, and it should be stressed that there is no possibility of producing a vaccine which can be used to immunize whole populations against cancer.

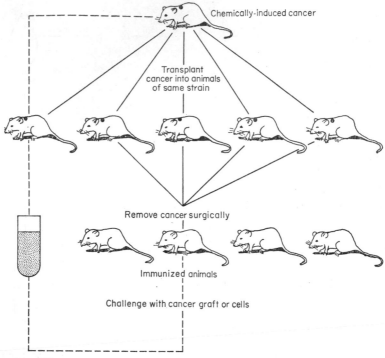

FIGURE 28

Showing how immunity can be produced against chemically-induced cancer when transplanted to normal compatible rats, and then surgically removed.

UNIQUENESS OF CANCER ANTIGENS

Cancers induced by chemical carcinogens have highly specific individual cancer antigens (Figure 29). That is, if an animal is immunized, by one of the methods outlined, against a particular cancer (C1) induced by a carcinogen (X), the immunity will only protect against this cancer C1. This means that another cancer (C2) induced by the same carcinogen (X) in an animal of the same strain and indistinguishable from C1 by the usual pathological methods will develop just as well in C1-immunized animals as in untreated animals. It has even been demonstrated, for example, that two cancers induced in one animal by injecting the carcinogen into different sites are immunologically different and induc-

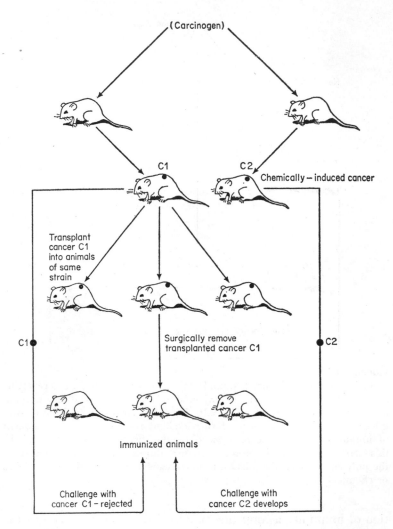

FIGURE 29

Showing that chemically-induced cancers possess individual cancer-specific antigens. Two cancers are induced by the same chemical carcinogen (X) in two rats of an inbred strain. One cancer C1 is transplanted into other rats of the same strain. These grafts develop and then are surgically removed. This results in the cancer C1-grafted rats developing immunity to cancer C1. These rats are not immune to the other Cancer (C2) and this develops as readily in the C1-immune rats as in normal rats.

105

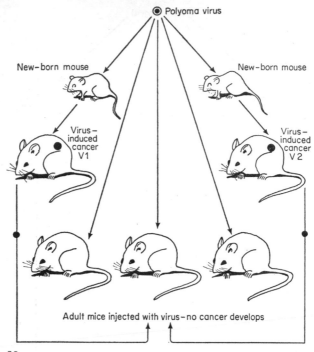

FIGURE 30

Shows how virus-induced animal cancers have common cancer-specific antigens. When polyoma virus is injected into new-born mice they develop polyoma-induced cancers (V1, V2). Polyoma virus injected into adult mice does not lead to cancer formation, but results in the development of immunity to the cancers induced by the virus in new-born mice. In this case, the resistance protects against almost all cancers induced by the polyoma virus in the mice, but not to cancers induced by other viruses or chemicals.

tion of immunity against one provided no protection against the other. These observations are of considerable importance in considering the possibility of immunotherapy of human cancer, since various assessments suggest that a high proportion, some put the figure as great as 80 per cent, are carcinogen-induced. This means that it would only be practicable to treat a patient, for example, by immunization with his own irradiated cancer cells, using tissue removed at surgery.

In sharp contrast to this individual antigenic specificity of chemically induced cancers, those induced by viruses have common cancer antigens (Figure 30). For instance, cancers can be induced at a multiplicity of sites in the mouse, including breast, skin and bone, following inoculation of new-born mice with polyoma virus (see p. 75). In this case, individual cancers are readily distinguishable by the usual pathological criteria, but induction of immunity to one cancer will confer on the host protection against almost all the other types induced by the same virus. Likewise leukaemia can be induced in mice with a number of viruses such as those discovered by Moloney, Rauscher and Gross. In each case, immunity to one type of leukaemia will protect against other leukaemias caused by the same viruses, but not to those induced by other viruses. The possibility of a viral aetiology for human cancers is, of course, still unproven. However, leukaemia and a special form of cancer occurring in African children (Burkitt lymphoma) are both thought to have a virus involvement. In these cases, it is feasible that each type may have common cancer-specific antigens as in the virus-induced animal cancers. From these considerations it may eventually be possible to develop more general methods for immunological treatment.

DISTRIBUTION OF CANCER ANTIGENS

Most virus-induced cancers possess cancer-specific antigens although there may be some differences in their antigenic activity. In the case of chemically-induced cancers, there are much greater differences in antigenic activity and it now appears that not all of these types carry cancer-specific antigens. For example, virtually all liver cancers induced by carcinogenic aminoazo dyes in the rat have cancer antigens which are effective in producing immunity. In contrast, cancers of the breast and liver produced in rats by another carcinogen, 2-acetylamino-fluorene, are only infrequently antigenic. The significance of these differences in antigenicity is still unknown although one explanation suggests that cancers which take a long time to develop may be deficient in specific antigens. These observations are of considerable importance when considering the significance of studies with experimental cancers in relation to the human disease, since they indicate the requirement of simple methods for detecting cancer specific antigens in selecting patients for treatment by immunological methods.

IMMUNITY TO CANCER IN THE ORIGINAL HOST

Although most investigations have been made using experimentally-induced cancers further transplanted in animals of the inbred strain of origin (cf. Figures 27 and 28), similar immunological reactions can be demonstrated in animals with primary cancers. When primary rat sarcomas, for example, are totally removed (and it is important that no malignant tissue is left behind), the rats reject a reinoculum of the same cancer which nevertheless grows in normal, untreated rats. This suggests that the primary host possessed a certain level of resistance to its own cancer but this was not sufficiently great to cause its rejection. There are several reasons for this, which may also explain why cancer cells, which are antigenically distinct, can develop in the first place. One obvious reason may be that the amount of antigen in the cancer cell is insufficient to produce a large enough immune response to kill off all the cancer cells which are replicating faster than normal cells. This is comparable to the situation where a bacterial infection cannot be suppressed solely by the body's immune reaction. In this case some other agent, such as an antibiotic, is needed to arrest bacterial growth until the host immunity can deal with the bacteria. Unfortunately most of the agents which can be used to kill cancer cells, such as radiotherapy or the various cancer chemotherapeutic drugs, also have the property of depressing immunological mechanisms. For this reason, some drugs originally developed as anti-cancer agents are now used specifically for immunosuppression in organ transplantation. Another feature which influences host reactivity against cancer cell antigens is the immunosuppressive action of the actual inducing agent, since many carcinogens, such as the polycyclic hydrocarbons, are immunosuppressive. Other factors such as the age and nutritional status of the host are also of importance in determining the immunological capacity of animals. Finally, in the systems where tumours are induced by virus in new-born animals or where the agent is present throughout the lifetime of the animal (mouse leukaemia), the immune system of the host is continuously exposed to large amounts of virally determined antigens and this will result in the development of 'tolerance' against these antigens. This is comparable to the situation already described (Figure 26) where inoculation of cells from one mouse strain into new-born mice of a second strain renders the recipients tolerant to the antigens on the injected cells.

HUMAN STUDIES AND THE IMPLICATIONS FOR CANCER TREATMENT

The reality of cancer-specific antigens is well established so far as experimentally induced animal cancers are concerned, and it is now feasible to consider the implications of laboratory data in the treatment of human cancer. To begin with there is evidence that immunological reactions occur against human cancer, although, because of the difficulties and ethical problems of human experimentation, this is less direct. For example, there are a number of established cases of spontaneous regression of cancer in man. Burkitt lymphomas occurring in African children can be cured in a number of cases following treatment with anti-cancer drugs and the degree of response suggests that immunological factors may be contributing to the treatment. Conversely there are reports of the sudden reappearance of a cancer after a long latent interval, often coinciding with treatments which are known to suppress the immunological system. This is also an attendant problem in organ transplantation and there are reports, fortunately rare, of patients with kidney grafts who, because they had to be maintained on immunosuppressive drugs to prevent rejection of the transplanted organs, developed cancer from malignant cells transferred with the kidney graft.

More direct evidence of host resistance to cancer has been provided in autotransplantation studies carried out in the USA. In these studies, cancer cells taken from a patient at operation and re-injected at another site were found not to develop in many cases. Such observations compare with the experimental studies on the resistance to re-implantation of rat cancer cells following total removal of the primary growth.

Accepting then that immune factors may be operative in human cancer, how best can immunotherapy be used? In the first place the marked variation in the antigenic activity of animal cancers indicates the necessity for methods to detect cancer-specific antigens in human material. In some experimental systems these antigens can be detected on the surface of cancer cells using a fluorescent antibody test (Figure 31). It should be explained that one of the responses produced by an antigen is the production of special proteins called antibodies, which circulate in the blood. The antibody proteins have the property of reacting only with the antigen which induced their production and in many cases, particularly in infectious diseases such as pneumonia, this is how immunity is mediated.

When animals are immunized against cancer cells as already described, the induction of resistance to the cancer is frequently accompanied by the production of antibodies which circulate in the blood. Although it is not thought that these antibodies play a significant role in cancer rejection, they are of particular value as indicators of tumour immunity, since they react specifically with cancer antigens on the cell surface. One way in which this

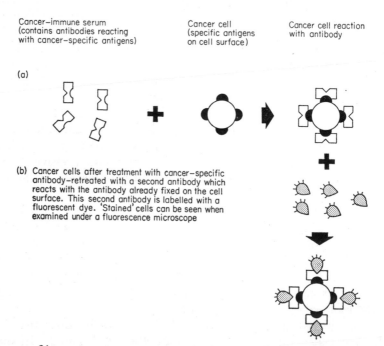

Cancer–immune serum (contains antibodies reacting with cancer–specific antigens)

Cancer cell (specific antigens on cell surface)

Cancer cell reaction with antibody

(a)

(b) Cancer cells after treatment with cancer–specific antibody–retreated with a second antibody which reacts with the antibody already fixed on the cell surface. This second antibody is labelled with a fluorescent dye. 'Stained' cells can be seen when examined under a fluorescence microscope

FIGURE 31

Fluorescent antibody technique for detecting antigen markers on cancer cells.

POSSIBLE METHODS FOR CANCER IMMUNOTHERAPY

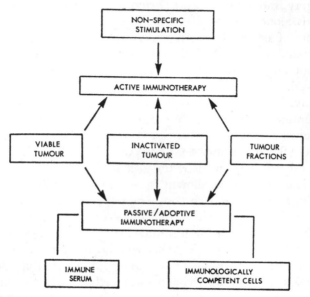

FIGURE 32

can be demonstrated involves 'staining' the cancer cells with antibody which is bound to a fluorescent dye (Figure 31). In this way, cancer cells can be shown specifically to bind these antibodies to the cell surface. Using this technique, cancer-specific antigens have been demonstrated on the cell surface in a number of experimental systems including virus-induced mouse leukaemia and chemically induced liver cancer. The technique is now proving to be of value in detecting cancer-specific reactions in man, particularly in the case of the Burkitt lymphoma in African children and probably also in human leukaemia. It is to be expected that further experimentation with techniques of this type will eventually make it possible to determine whether or not other types of human cancer carry cancer-specific antigens.

Given the situation when a human cancer can be shown to have cancer-specific antigens, the findings from animal experimentation suggest various ways in which these may be brought into play in the treatment of the disease (Figure 32). These must be considered together with conventional forms of therapy such as surgery, radiotherapy and chemotherapy since immunological methods alone are not likely to be efficient in destroying large numbers of cancer cells. In experimental studies, for example, the maximum levels of immunity obtained can cause rejection of about one million cells and in some cases fewer still can be destroyed.

Firstly, it may be possible to stimulate, in a non-specific way, the immune reaction already produced by the patient against his own cancer. This may be achieved by administering agents such as BCG (Bacille Calmette Guerin) which is a non-virulent form of the tubercle bacillus used for vaccination against tuberculosis. Preliminary trials have shown, for example, that BCG treatment following conventional chemotherapy produces long periods of remission in patients with leukaemia. Another possibility yet to be fully explored is active immunization against cancer antigens. As in experimental studies, this will be most practicable with cancer cells inactivated in some manner, to ensure that the treatment does not transfer living cancer cells to other parts of the body resulting in 'secondary' growths. This form of therapy may be used to enhance immune reactions following other forms of treatment, so as to eliminate small numbers of residual cancer cells. Also, the observation that re-implantation of a small piece of a primary animal cancer inactivated by X-irradiation makes the primary growth more sensitive to radiotherapy suggests that this treatment may also be used as an adjuvant to other forms of therapy. Only within the last year has it become possible to isolate cancer antigens in an active form and at present the separation methods are relatively crude. Eventually, however, it should be possible to isolate cancer antigens in a relatively pure state and this may provide safer and more efficient material for immunization therapy.

An alternative approach to the immunological treatment of cancer is by passive immunization, that is, transfer of immunity from another host. In classical situations such as infectious diseases, this is carried out by the injection of serum antibodies (antiserum) prepared by immunizing another species with the antigens. For example tetanus antitoxin prepared by immunizing horses with tetanus toxin is used for protection against tetanus. As already mentioned, serum antibodies are not usually effective in transferring immunity to cancer cells in experimental animal systems. On the contrary, in many cases, treatment of cancer cells with serum from animals immunized against the cancer actually protects these cells and thus enhances cancer growth. This finding of so-called enhancing antibodies is common to almost all situations involving transplantation of tissues, and is one reason why clinicians have been cautious in attempting to apply immunological methods to the treatment of cancer patients. Clearly, therefore, treatment of cancer with immune sera is not yet a practical procedure.

In experimental cancer studies, passive transfer of immunity has been obtained using not serum, but the so-called lymphoid cells obtained from a variety of sources such as blood (white cells), lymph nodes and spleen. These 'immune-cells' are frequently highly efficient in this respect and in some cases a ratio as low as four immune cells to one cancer cell is sufficient to prevent growth. The situation in man is much more complicated because unlike inbred animals, two individuals (unless they are identical twins) are genetically different. Therefore, when lymphoid cells, which are themselves competent to produce an immune reaction (i.e. so-called immunologically competent cells), are transferred from the immunized donor to the recipient cancer patient, they will attack not only the cancer cells but also other cells in the recipient. Nevertheless trials with this sort of immunotherapy have been carried out in the USA using white cells isolated from the blood of an individual immunized against another patient's cancer. Injecting these white cells back into the cancer donor produced some positive effects in a number of cases and two patients had complete remissions for at least two years. Much still remains to be discovered about the mechanism of action of the transferred lymphoid cells. Recently methods have been developed whereby this immunity can be transferred using an isolated ribonucleic acid fraction from the cells which contains their 'immune information', thereby avoiding unwanted attack on normal cells.

Cancer immunology has made enormous advances during the past decade and is now at the threshold of discovering how resistance to cancer can be produced and transmitted. For the present, advances must be made with caution since, as with all unknowns, the procedures are not without hazards. At least, however, the problems can be seen and it is only a matter of time and hard work before the ideas are translated into facts.

CHAPTER V

CANCER AND MAN'S ENVIRONMENT

R. W. BALDWIN and J. Q. MATTHIAS

Man has been engaged in a continuous struggle for survival with the hostile animate and inanimate forces present in his natural environment since the dawn of existence. In contrast, however, to the relatively stable environment of the past, changes today are ever more frequent and more profound. During the last 150 years, man has become increasingly exposed to new chemical and physical hazards. The dangers from coal-tar, soot and oil, and the aromatic amines of the dyestuffs and rubber industries have already been described.

Experimentally, a single exposure to some carcinogens can initiate a malignant change, but generally speaking continued exposure leads to both a higher incidence of cancers and to their earlier development. A co-carcinogen can enhance the carcinogenic activity of a known carcinogen. The importance of co-carcinogens (which are not carcinogenic *per se*) is not known in human cancer, but in animals carcinogenesis appears to occur in two stages: firstly, tumour initiation; and secondly, tumour promotion. Tumour initiators alter tissues permanently in the direction of tumour formation, but do not lead to actual development of tumours themselves, while promoters take initiated tissues, but not normal tissues, forward to the stage of tumour formation. Both may be acting together or a long interval may separate exposure to the initiator and to the promoter. If *one* substance acts both as the initiator and the promoter it is known as a complete carcinogen. Tumour promotion, unlike tumour initiation, is a reversible process. The role of tumour promoters in man is extremely difficult to clarify but, should it prove of importance, then the implications will be considerable in view of the reversibility of the process. There is little doubt about the wisdom of reducing exposure to any possible carcinogen as much as is practicable. Statistical data suggest, for example, that the risk of developing lung cancer is less in persons who stop smoking; evidence which favours the belief that cigarette smoke is a co-carcinogen rather than a complete carcinogen, the effect of which would be irreversible *(vide infra)*. Of particular danger are insidious and long-delayed effects resulting from prolonged exposure to small or even minute amounts of some carcinogen : not infrequently tumours declare themselves many years after exposure has ceased.

The interval between exposure to a carcinogenic agent and the development of the tumour (the latent interval) may be as short as five to seven years or as long as the life span. There is always a minimal latent period, despite massive repeated exposure. There is always, therefore, some period in which it is possible that some counter measures might succeed in preventing the development of the cancer, or at least in postponing the event. Not uncommonly, entirely unsuspected cancers are found at post-mortem examination. Clearly such information is of vital importance epidemiologically in assessing cause and effect. Serious consideration must be given to ways of increasing the proportion of examinations after death which are carried out in Great Britain.

FOOD

Man encounters potentially carcinogenic substances in every part of his environment.

Chemicals such as herbicides, insecticides, fertilizers, anti-biotics, detergents, metals, and the products of fungi and moulds contaminate his food.

The potential contribution of the latter are particularly well illustrated by the story of the aflatoxins.

In the late 1950s poultry breeders became seriously alarmed by a marked rise in a liver disease in turkeys termed Turkey X, and in 1960 some 100,000 young turkeys were lost. The cause of the disease was traced to the use of a consignment of Brazilian groundnuts in the mashes used for feeding. These nuts were con-taminated by a mould called *Aspergillus flavus*. Subsequently toxic factors (aflatoxins) produced by the mould were isolated and some of these substances have proved to be carcinogenic in several animal species. Aflatoxins, as the name implies, are highly poisonous; trace amounts are sufficient to kill young ducklings within a few days. Other species such as rats and mice are less sensitive to the immediate toxic action of aflatoxins but in many cases, they later develop liver and kidney cancer. It is of interest that the aflatoxins are totally different in chemical nature from other chemical carcinogens which induce liver cancer (Figure 33) and these observations have prompted a much wider search for new types of carcinogens amongst mould products and other naturally occurring substances.

There is no direct evidence as yet that aflatoxins are carcinogenic for man but, at least in this situation, the observation of

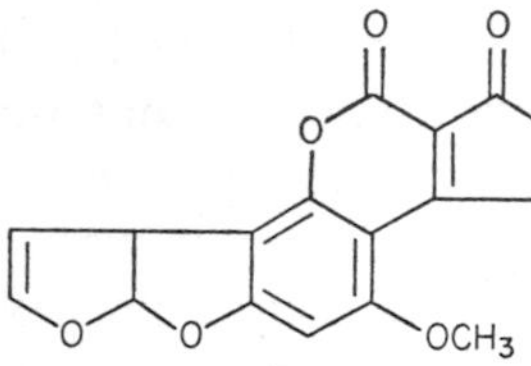

Aflatoxin B
(*Aspergillus flavus* strain)

FIGURE 33

cancer in exposed animals provides a guideline for human studies. For instance, it has been suggested that the high incidence of liver cancer in Africa and the Far East may result from exposure to naturally occurring carcinogens in diet. This observation, in turn, raises the possibility that these natural carcinogens may be aflatoxins or some other mould products arising from contamination of inadequately stored foodstuffs. Fortunately, official health organizations are now well aware of this possibility because of the much greater facility for interchange of information through organisations such as the International Union Against Cancer. There is therefore a real possibility of effecting preventative measures.

In addition to (unknown) contaminants, (known) food additives of increasing complexity are now used as colouring or flavouring agents, artificial sweeteners, preservatives and emulsifying agents. Stringent tests are required in this country before such substances may be incorporated into foods and it is fairly certain that no *potent* carcinogens are introduced. Another source of food con-

117

tamination occurs via trace residues of the insecticides or herbicides used agriculturally. For example, certain insecticides such as aldrin, dieldrin and DDT are unfortunately highly stable and so are absorbed into animal fat and by this means are incorporated into human foods. At present the level of exposure to these substances is well below the maximum daily intake levels recommended by the WHO Expert Committee on Pesticide Residues, but the possibility of a health hazard certainly exists and needs to be controlled. Apart from chemicals deliberately introduced into foods there are other contaminants that may arise from storage or processing. The cause of outbreaks of severe liver disease in sheep in Norway was traced to the consumption of fish meal which had been preserved with sodium nitrite. The fish meal was later shown to be contaminated with a potent carcinogen, dimethylnitrosamine, presumably formed by reaction of dimethylamine, produced during slight decomposition of the fish, with the sodium nitrite used as preservative. Dimethylnitrosamine is highly toxic in many species and induces both liver damage and eventually liver cancer.

Not all toxic substances in foods are artificially induced, and the discovery of a toxic mould product, aflatoxin, has already been described. Since it has been estimated that there may be as many as 250,000 different species of fungi in Nature, it is highly likely that other cancer-producing mould products will be discovered as a result of further studies.

CARCINOGENIC HAZARDS FROM DRUGS

The decision to allow or disallow a substance for human use is not always clear cut, but must depend upon a consideration of its potential value in other situations. For instance, many drugs by design are toxic substances. Under these circumstances, evaluation of the cancer risk that may arise in the therapeutic use of a drug involves an assessment of the balance between benefit to the patient and the overall cancer risk during life expectancy. In simple terms, there is no logic in excluding a drug because it may produce a carcinogenic response sometime in the future if, by so doing, patients deprived of its beneficial effects die from other diseases long before this time. For example, preparations containing a complex of iron and dextran are of considerable value in the treatment of iron-deficiency anaemia. These complexes have also been found to induce cancer in animals so that their continued therapeutic use is open to question. Certain recommendations can readily be made such as withdrawal from use in young patients and especially pregnant women. Since, however, the latent period for cancer induction in man is likely to be more than fifteen to twenty years, it is justifiable to continue their use in older patients whose life expectancy is less than this.

LUNG CANCER

During the past fifty years, lung cancer has changed from being an infrequent to a major cause of death, particularly in males. This trend is international, lung cancer death rates rising to a greater or lesser extent in many countries with the British Isles now at the top of the list (Figure 34). According to the recent Annual Report of the Chief Medical Officer of the Ministry of Health on the state of Public Health, deaths from lung cancer in Britain in 1967 totalled 28,252, of which 23,548 were males and

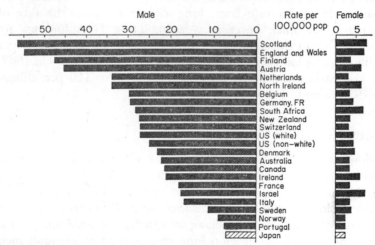

FIGURE 34

Lung cancer death rates (1956–57) in various countries. [From W. C. Hueper, 'Occupational and Environmental Cancers of the Respiratory System', *Recent Results in Cancer Research*, **3** (1966), Springer-Verlag, Heidelberg.]

119

only 4,704 were females. Moreover nearly two-thirds of the increase in total deaths from cancer between 1966 and 1967 could be accounted for by a rise in deaths from lung cancer. We have now reached the position where almost four times as many people die from lung cancer each year as are killed in motor-vehicle accidents.

This phenomenal rise in lung cancer is in striking contrast to the current trend for most other forms of human cancer, where the incidence over the past few years has shown little change or in some cases, has even declined. For instance, deaths from lung cancer in the USA have risen steadily over the years from a level of below 5 per 100,000 of the male population in 1930, and by 1965 the incidence at 40 per 100,000 men was eight times greater (Figure 35). During the same thirty-five year period, the incidence of cancer of the stomach fell from about 30 to 10 per 100,000 of the male population, whilst cancer at other sites such as colon and prostate showed little change in incidence. In comparison with the situation in men, the death rate for cancer of the stomach in women also showed a slight decrease over the same thirty-five year period. Other types of cancer also showed only slight changes in incidence, but contrary to the catastrophic rise in the death rate from lung cancer in men, the rate of increase was much lower in women. These USA findings are comparable to the situation in Britain where the death rate per million living has risen in males from 784 in 1958 to 999 in 1967. In comparison the death rates in females were 119 per million in 1958 rising to 189 in 1967.

OCCUPATIONAL FACTORS

To what then may this phenomenal rise in lung cancer be attributed? Industry-associated lung cancer, like bladder cancer in dyestuff workers, has been demonstrated in many cases by epidemiological studies. For instance over 100 years ago, it was shown that miners of Schneeberg and Jachymor were thirty-three times more liable to develop lung cancer than other adult men in Vienna, possibly due to exposure to radioactive ores. There is also epidemiological evidence that the risk of lung cancer is very high in asbestos workers and the problems of asbestos exposure and the biological effects of this material are quite rightly

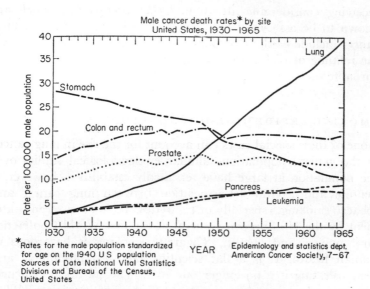

Male cancer death rates* by site
United States, 1930—1965

*Rates for the male population standardized
for age on the 1940 U S population
Sources of Data National Vital Statistics
Division and Bureau of the Census,
United States

Epidemiology and statistics dept.
American Cancer Society, 7—67

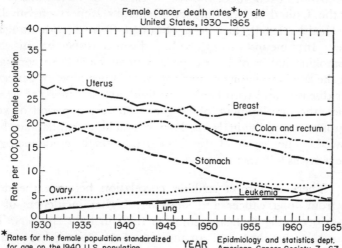

Female cancer death rates* by site
United States, 1930—1965

*Rates for the female population standardized
for age on the 1940 U S population
Sources of Data National Vital Statistics
Division and Bureau of the Census,
United States

Epidmiology and statistics dept.
American Cancer Society, 7—67

FIGURE 35

Comparison of cancer death rates by site in males and females in USA between the years 1930 and 1965. [Reprinted from *J. Am. Med. Assoc.* **203**, 34 (1968).]

receiving considerable attention. Other occupations which are known to be associated with unusually high incidences of lung cancer include work involving exposure to radioactive substances, the refining of nickel and the manufacture of bichromates from chromite ores.

SMOKING—EPIDEMIOLOGICAL STUDIES

None of these special cases can account for the rise in lung cancer in the general population. Similar epidemiological studies over the population at large have repeatedly established, however, a definite and irrefutable association between lung cancer and tobacco smoking, especially of cigarettes. To quote a recent statement by the US Surgeon General at the first World Conference on Smoking and Health, 'Cigarette smoking is hazardous to human health. It is a flat scientific fact. Establishing it and demonstrating it is no longer our goal.' The statistical evidence, summarized in reports of the Royal College of Physicians (1962) and the United States Surgeon General's Report on Smoking and Health (1964), has been obtained from a wide range of surveys. In some instances these have been retrospective, in which the smoking habits of lung cancer patients have been compared with the smoking habits of patients with other types of cancer or other diseases, and with healthy individuals. In other *prospective* studies, the development of lung cancer over a period of years in groups of individuals of known smoking habits has been followed. The essential findings from these epidemiological surveys are as follows :

1. There is a most striking correlation between the death rate from lung cancer and smoking; higher incidences of the disease occurring in heavy smokers than in light smokers. This means that the chance of an individual developing lung cancer is directly proportional to the number of cigarettes smoked each day and the duration of the smoking habit.

2. Lung cancer rates in communities where smoking is prohibited, e.g. Seventh-Day Adventists, are very much lower than in neighbouring permissive communities.

3. Prospective surveys in groups where there has been a decrease in cigarette consumption show a corresponding decrease

in lung cancer incidence. For instance, the lung cancer death rate in a large group of British male doctors, many of whom have stopped smoking in recent years, has fallen by about 30 per cent in the ten-year period 1954 to 1964. During the same overall period, the lung cancer rate in the general population increased and it is now almost 2½ times as great as that in doctors. These studies also show that lung cancer is potentially preventable and the mortality from this disease would be strikingly reduced in the long term if cigarette smoking was to stop.

4. The dramatic rise in lung cancer observed in males has not yet been so great in females (Figure 36). This may be explained by the fact that fewer women smoked, at least not on any large scale, until around the 1930s. That is, there is something like a 30 to 35-year time lag in the exposure to the harmful effects of cigarette smoking and the development of lung cancer. If this interpretation should prove to be correct, it follows that unless smoking habits change, the dreadful possibility has to be faced of female mortality from lung cancer rising within the next ten to twenty years.

SMOKING—EXPERIMENTAL STUDIES

At the experimental level, many studies are being carried out to isolate and identify cancer-inducing substances in tobacco

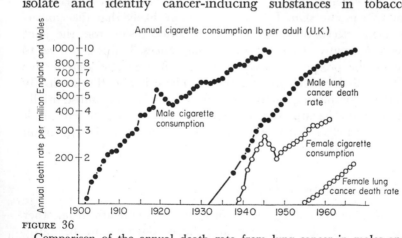

FIGURE 36

Comparison of the annual death rate from lung cancer in males and females with the rate of consumption of tobacco. [From Eng. 96/703, 1968, HMSO, London.]

123

smoke. The present position is that tobacco smoke, condensed by passing through a cold trap, will induce cancer when repeatedly applied to the skin of mice and rabbits or injected into the lungs of rats. Efforts to induce lung cancer in animals by inhalation of tobacco smoke have not been entirely successful, but it should be realized that the lung structure of small animals such as mice is quite different from that of humans. Nevertheless the induction of malignant lung cancer in mice exposed throughout their lives to tobacco smoke was reported in 1967 and these studies lay the foundation for the experimental verification of the epidemiological findings.

Much attention has also been given towards identifying chemical carcinogens in tobacco smoke. This has resulted in the identification of literally dozens of compounds which have known cancer-inducing properties or which have the property of accelerating the action of carcinogens (co-carcinogens or promoters). Most of these are only present at low concentrations and so the carcinogenic action of tobacco smoke concentrates in experimental tests such as mouse skin cancer-induction cannot be accounted for by single constituents. For example, whilst one of the most potent polycyclic hydrocarbon carcinogens, 3, 4-benzopyrene has been detected in tobacco smoke concentrates, the concentration of this carcinogen was much too low to account for the carcinogenic activity of the tobacco smoke concentrate towards mouse skin. It now seems more likely that the cancer-inducing effects of tobacco-smoke products result from the joint action of many of the constituent substances. If this is proved to be so, the prospect of developing a 'safe cigarette' or effective filters will be much more difficult. There is also the possibility that the promoting factors in tobacco smoke may substantially increase the hazard from carcinogens present in polluted air; it is well established that lung cancer mortality is higher in urban than in rural areas.

SMOKING AND HEALTH

In addition to the lung cancer problems, many deaths from other diseases such as bronchitis and heart disease can be fairly attributed to smoking. It has been reported, for example, that amongst males aged thirty-five to forty-forty years, the heavy smoker is nearly ten times more likely to have fatal coronary heart disease. Despite these now well established relationships between health hazards and cigarette smoking, little impact has been made on the overall consumption of cigarettes, or on the number of smokers. The reasons for this are complex, but one obvious factor has been the willingness of the public to accept the risk of developing lung cancer despite all the evidence. According to a recent survey in the United States, about 75 per cent of smokers interviewed accepted that smoking is a hazard to health. Against this there is some evidence of a discernible decrease in cigarette consumption but there would appear to be a little hope in the immediate future of obtaining a complete discontinuation of smoking amongst the public. Consequently, a greater effort is needed to broadcast the facts to the community and to provide a proper counselling service to those who desire to stop smoking. Current expenditure by the Government on health education in regard to smoking is now of the order of £100,000 per annum although this is supplemented to some extent by the expenditure of local health authorities. The inadequacy of this programme is revealed when compared with the enormous expenditure in the United Kingdom on commercial advertising of cigarettes, tobacco and smokers' requisites, which was estimated to total £11,000,000 in 1960. Much more also needs to be learned about the 'whys' of smoking in order properly to advise against the habit. In a recent survey in the USA amongst 9,000 smokers, it was estimated that about 10 per cent used smoking as a stimulant to help wake up and feel more alert and about 8 per cent derived pleasure from the physical manipulation of the cigarette (holding, twisting, flicking ash). Only about one-third derived a positive effect such as pleasure or relaxation whilst a further 40 to 45 per cent used cigarettes to decrease negative feelings such as depression. These findings certainly indicate the necessity for categorizing smokers according to the needs which smoking fulfils in attempting to advise them how to abandon the habit.

The gravity of the danger which smoking presents to health cannot be stressed too much. The abolition of cigarette smoking could reduce Britain's death rate by one-tenth, and the saving in terms of disability and loss of working capacity would be even greater. This is a situation which effects every individual, man, woman and even child; the community must be encouraged by

125

every means possible to come to terms with the habit of smoking. Many people believe that filter-tipped cigarettes are safer and this is one reason for the great increase in their popularity. It should be stressed that, even though there are general arguments in favour of tipped cigarettes, the safety of any filter available is unproven. Indeed some produce little or no appreciable reduction in the tar and nicotine content of cigarette smoke and as such may be positively harmful in producing a false sense of security. At the present time, therefore, there is no such thing as a 'safe cigarette' and the only sound advice that can be given to the smoker who cannot give up the habit is to change to pipe or cigar. The ultimate aim should nevertheless be to discourage the habit of smoking since all available evidence indicates that *to stop smoking is to reduce the risks*.

RADIATION

The incidence of malignant disease (in particular leukaemia) is increased by exposure to ionizing radiation. Regardless of whether it is a primary or only a secondary factor, at present the only means by which the incidence can be reduced is by limiting exposure. Current information suggests, however, that less than 1 per cent of leukaemias could be caused by radiation from diagnostic procedures. The human foetus is especially sensitive and it has been accepted that radiological pelvimetry can produce a 40 per cent increase in the foetal risk of malignancy. It must be emphasized that even this means that less than 1 in 1,000 babies so exposed would be expected to develop cancer. Nevertheless malignant disease accounts for 1 in 5 of all deaths before the age of fifteen in this country. Some cancers are virtually only found in children or adolescents and there is little doubt that many are initiated *in utero*. It is not possible to decide whether obstetric radiology, which is usually undertaken towards the end of pregnancy, has operated as an initiating or promoting factor : neither, of course, is it possible to assess the teratogenic effect of chemicals (many in the form of drugs) or viruses. It is noteworthy that the greatest risk of incurring recognizable congenital defects is in early pregnancy when the rapid formation of new cell lines constitutes a special risk. Apart from certain obvious examples (Mongolism with a thirty times increased risk of developing leukaemia) childhood cancers are seldom associated with recognizable congenital defects, suggesting perhaps that the first event in the chain of cancer induction is inconspicuous and capable of affecting a single gene without producing other obvious effects.

Studies are under way to discover whether recently introduced improvements in radiological techniques, in particular image intensification resulting in dose reductions of some twenty times, have succeeded in reducing or eliminating cancers due to diagnostic radiation procedures. In any event, no diagnostic procedure should be advised without good reason. Every effort should be made to reduce the dose of radiation given and pregnancy must be excluded before carrying out radiological investigations involving irradiation of the abdomen in women of child-bearing age. It must be remembered that the employment of X-rays and radioactive chemicals for the diagnosis of disease are of incalculable value and that to date, other than in pregnancy, no demonstrable links have been established between diagnostic irradiation and cancer hazard to the patient.

The introduction of remote relay television techniques has reduced the hazard for those working in the field of diagnostic radiography and in industry, where radioactive techniques for controlling many aspects of production are becoming ever more common. Radiation is also used for treating benign as well as malignant conditions and undoubtedly, as such, is responsible for inducing some cancers. Clearly radiotherapy confers overwhelming advantages in the treatment of malignant disease but strict care should be exercised in treating non-malignant conditions. There is general awareness of the risk of irradiating the neck region of children. The younger the patient when irradiated, the greater the probability of inducing cancer of the thyroid. There is also a recognized definite risk to treating ankylosing spondylitis with high doses. Small amounts of radioactivity are widely used in adults both for diagnostic purposes and for treatment. The doses are strictly controlled and the effects are carefully assessed. Nevertheless constant vigilance and reappraisal is necessary and possible harm balanced against the benefits conferred.

The testing of nuclear weapons in the atmosphere causes radioactive material to be dispersed over the whole world. It is still too early to be certain that it does not constitute a danger but, as a result of the 1963 Partial Test Ban Treaty, levels are expected to fall, and in any event they have never been high enough to justify altering the distribution and care of food.

VIRUSES

It has long been known that many tumours in animals (from fish to mammals) may be induced by viruses (p. 73). So far, however, no viruses have been isolated which are known to cause cancer in man.

The most common types of cancer occur in increasing frequency with age. The exceptions are tumours in organs associated with reproduction which are more common during the reproductive phase of life. In contrast are certain tumours of children which rarely occur in later years, such as Burkitt's tumour, lymphoblastic leukaemia and tumours of embryonal tissue. The pattern of incidence of the adult cancers fits in well with the mutational theory of carcinogesis which proposes that malignant mutations are in fact induced commonly by a variety of means (chemical, mechanical, radiation, etc.). It is envisaged that the undesirable abnormalities which arise are ordinarily eliminated by immunological means. However, with increasing age and diminishing immunological competence, the chances of a cancer developing become greater. The childhood tumours on the other hand could perhaps be explained as the result of infection with an oncogenic virus.

Some viruses are only capable of causing tumours if introduced into the immature animal. At birth most mammals have only very poorly developed immunological systems so that the virus itself or the cell containing the virus would tend not to be rejected. A state known as 'immunological tolerance' (p. 100) develops in which injected cells are no longer regarded, and dealt with, as foreign by the body but accepted as normal body cells. If this is so, then the active and passive measures usually employed to control virus infections will prove difficult to implement. Possibly some other approach will be necessary such as the prior stimulation of the mother's immune system. Nevertheless, although experimentally protection is more effective if inoculation is given before the virus, some protection occurs if given later, although it is usually proportionally less complete the nearer the end of the latent interval. Even if cancers are the result of a combination of viral and chemical factors, control of infection would be expected to reduce the incidence of tumours.

Alternatively since transformation of cells by oncogenic viruses gives rise to new antigens it may be possible to direct the attacks against these tumour antigens rather than against the virus as such.

Some oncogenic viruses also seem to find it more difficult to establish themselves after prior inoculation with relatively benign viruses such as herpes virus. Possibly some portal of entry or metabolic pathway is blocked, or alternatively the combination is eliminated immunologically. Perhaps in similar fashion, chemicals may eventually lead to the elimination of oncogenic virus. The success of thiosemicarbazone in the prevention of small-pox holds out hope that drugs may be developed capable of preventing possible virus-induced cancers in man.

Nucleic acids of viruses code for enzymes which sometimes are *unique* to the virus-infected cells, but in other cases are identical with pre-existing host enzymes differing only in quantity. It will almost certainly be possible to develop ways and means of inhibiting any *unique enzymes*. However, enzymes not lending themselves to specific chemical attack because of actual qualitative differences could perhaps still be vulnerable by virtue of their increased concentration.

Viruses known to be oncogenic in certain animals may contaminate live viruses used to protect man against other diseases such as poliomyelitis, measles and yellow fever. Such hazards, now theoretical, may achieve practical importance in the future. The greatest potential hazard is in the very young. On present evidence, the benefits from vaccinations far outweigh the theoretical dangers from contamination with oncogenic viruses. No increased risks have been demonstrated in adults or in research workers handling large inocula of animal tumour viruses, despite the appearance of specific antibodies in their serum. In addition, deliberate infection has failed to produce tumours in man. However, as in the case of potential chemical carcinogens, the sensible appreciation of possible risks and methods of avoiding or reducing them are the responsibility of all involved in experimental work using oncogenic viruses.

Clearly, before any of the discoveries relating to virus-induced tumours in animals can be applied to cancer prevention in man, viruses oncogenic for man must be identified. Viruses isolated from human tumours so far are thought to be inconsequential 'super-added passengers' or 'secondary invaders' rather than 'inducers'. However, as viruses may be so closely integrated into the cells as to be non-infective and virtually to defy identification by present-day methods, there remains the very distinct possibility that viruses may play some part in the development of at least some tumours in man. The geographical and climatic distribution, the familial coincidence and seasonal variations of some cancers suggests infective factors. Possibly in certain cases viruses, or virus-like genetic material is transmitted to the very young or to the non-immune by insects. In Britain, animals could well form reservoirs for such agents. Lymphosarcoma (and leucosis) is one of the commoner forms of cancer in cats, dogs, cattle and birds, and is almost certainly of viral aetiology. The possibility that transmissible agents in human breast cancer have a role to play comparable to the Bittner virus of mice must also be seriously entertained. If some forms of human cancer are caused by specific viruses, and not by some chance event in the genetic apparatus of the cell, the possibility of evolving effective preventive measures greatly increases. It is not going to be easy to gather information on the means of transmission from one person to another. Probably the best hope lies in the possibility of a specific cancer, such as acute lymphoblastic leukaemia of children, having much in common with the animal equivalent. It must be stressed however that at the present time there is no evidence which suggests that human leukaemia is in any way connected with animal leukaemia. However, if ways and means can be found of preventing spontaneous leukaemia in animals some of them might be applicable to man. Amongst the possibilities are:

1.   Breaking the cycle of transmission.
     (a) from one person to another (horizontal and vertical).
     (b) from animals to man.
2.   The administration of vaccines
     (a) Passive (serum, containing antibodies):
         (i) specific to the individual tumour.
         (ii) non-specific – may be valuable during the first few

days or weeks of life or administered to the mother during pregnancy.

(b) Active :

(i) specific, using attenuated virus or purified preparations of the new antigens induced by the virus.

(ii) non-specific stimulation of the immune mechanisms to raise general resistance.

3. The development of anti-viral drugs.

It is perhaps in the isolation of new cell antigens, induced by the oncogenic virus, from malignant tissue or from tissue cultures infected with the virus that the greatest hope lies. Such a vaccine of itself would not cause cancer and by hyperstimulating a competent immunological system could well achieve the degree of control necessary to contain or destroy transformed cells.

GENETIC FACTORS

It is possible by inbreeding to produce strains in which every animal develops a particular type of cancer. The nearest equivalent in man is familial polyposis of the colon and rectum, and the skin condition xeroderma pigmentosum where eventual malignant changes are virtually inevitable. In the first instance, apparently no additional carcinogenic agent is necessary but in the second it is thought that ultra-violet light may act as a co-carcinogen.

Other than these obvious examples, many cancers run in families. The genetic information regarding malignancy is presumably transmitted from parent to progeny directly in the DNA of the chromosomes of the germ cell. In other instances the fundamental changes in the DNA may be imprinted as an acquired feature before fertilization or subsequently during development. For example, many chemicals and viruses are known to be capable of crossing the so-called placental barrier with comparative ease. Other means of access to the child include, infection taking place directly either at the time of delivery or subsequently, perhaps for example in the maternal milk.

The transmission of the initiating factor in the various ways outlined above would all tend to give the appearances of being inherited, although the mechanisms are clearly different. Vertically transmitted viruses acquiring access to the DNA by these various means might be of vital importance as primary (initiating) causes of malignant change. Unfortunately they are going to be anything but easy to detect. Present techniques are not sensitive enough in many instances to allow us to demonstrate the virus even in animal tumours which are known to be the result of infections with oncogenic viruses. In these cases it is suspected that the virus has become incorporated within the host's own genetic material, so that the substitutions can only be recognized by precise analysis of the strands of DNA.

CHROMOSOME ABNORMALITIES

The older the mother the greater the chance of her child developing abnormalities of the chromosomes whilst in utero. One such abnormality is known as trisomy 21 (3 instead of 2 chromosomes Number 21). As a result the child is a mongol and as such has a thirty times greater risk of developing leukaemia than a normal child. Other cancers are also more common in the offspring of older mothers. The increased risk is calculated at 40 per cent for children (other than mongols) of mothers over the age of forty compared with under twenty. While every encouragement should be given to women to have their families while they themselves are young, there is, however, no question of advising older women not to have children on account of increased cancer risks, for even if the risk was increased by 50 per cent this would amount to no more than 1 extra case for every 2,000 children !

Irradiation, viruses and chemicals are all known to produce visible chromosomal abnormalities. The damage may be so severe as to prevent the cell dividing successfully ever again and as such is self-limiting. However, damage of lesser degree may result in abnormal cells capable of further division and of passing the acquired abnormality on to future generations of cells. It is conceivable that a deficiency in genetic information necessary for the control of growth might be passed on; the new cell line would then possess one of the characteristics of malignancy, namely the ability to go on dividing.

Chromosomal changes, sufficiently crude to be recognized by

current methods, occur in malignant disease. In a minority of instances they are characteristic of the particular malignancy and can be recognized before the disease presents clinically. A classical example is that of the Philadelphia chromosome in chronic myelogenous leukaemia. It is not known how long the abnormality can be detected before the disease declares itself, but clearly the discovery opens up an entirely new field in the early diagnosis of cancer. There is no reason to doubt that the recognition of abnormalities in the chromosomes will become of vital importance in screening programmes both in the early diagnosis of the malignant state and in the recognition of precursor stages. Progress is hampered by the complex and time-consuming nature of the techniques presently available. New and precise ways of making detailed chemical and structural maps of the chromosome are urgently required.

Carcinogenic factors with weak effects are likely to be missed without special epidemiological surveys. Serious attempts must be made to throw light on possible causes by all means including the careful examination and investigation of every case of cancer and the elucidation of any possible environmental factors past and present, domestic and industrial, by questionnaire and interrogation. It may be hoped that the analysis of large numbers of patients suffering from similar types of cancer the world over will lead to the discovery of causative factors. Efforts to detect carcinogens in the environment, which in all possibility cause the developed disease in only 1 in 1,000 persons exposed, will be slow. It will be painstaking and demanding work of infinite complexity for which the public should be asked to give understanding and support. The more the man in the street knows about cancer the greater the chance that causal associations will be recognized.

CHAPTER VI

THE ROLE OF SURGERY IN THE MANAGEMENT OF CANCER

JOHN BRUCE

From the earliest recorded times, the removal or the physical destruction of obvious growths and excrescences on the human body has been a natural and a rational surgical exercise. Thus ablation by arsenical unguents is mentioned in the Ebers Papyrus, the earliest medical text from ancient Egypt; and Celsus, a Roman surgeon of the opening decades of the Christian era, was recommending removal of the breast by a method revived not long ago in one of our great London hospitals. Nearer home, Guy de Chauliac, the famous French surgeon at the beginning of the fourteenth century, advocated a combination of scalpel excision and a caustic application – zinc chloride – which is still in use for some cancers in the world famous Cancer Memorial Hospital in New York.

Until comparatively recently, then, cancer was almost entirely the province of the surgeon (or possibly of the quack, a breed unfortunately not yet extinct!). The challenge to the surgeon was to remove the growth and its obvious extensions, preferably and if possible without damage to the patient; and the history of cancer surgery has been of a search for better and more complete methods of so doing. Today the increasing longevity of our fellow citizens ensures that a not inconsiderable part of the work of the contemporary surgeon is devoted to treatment of malignant disease; but there have been important changes in surgical philosophy, status and practice. The objective of the surgeon is no longer only to remove cancerous tissues; he has a role – an important role – in prevention and in diagnosis as well in treatment.

Furthermore, he is no longer alone in the attack on malignant disease. Fifty years ago there was nothing other than operation to offer the cancer victim. Today there are other weapons of varying degrees of potency, and their use as an alternative to excisional surgery, or their deployment before, during and after operation have brought into the van colleagues who are skilled in these other tools and techniques. This does not imply a spirit of competition. Such methods are complementary to surgery, just as surgery is sometimes complementary to other methods, as for instance when an amputation is performed after an intensive course of irradiation for certain tumours of bone. There may have been a time when a charge of both pride and prejudice could have been levelled against both the surgeon and his 'rivals', but this is now a thing of the past; and the management of cancer is now a splendidly co-operative effort.

Furthermore, even in the field of strictly surgical endeavour, the individual surgeon often can no longer afford to plough a lone furrow. The growth of regional specialization makes it desirable or even imperative for one surgeon to seek the collaboration of others in special fields. The general surgeon may need the help of the plastic surgeon, the otolaryngologist may have to turn to the general surgeon, and so on. Malignant disease does not confine its ravages to the precise geographical territories into which modern surgery has disintegrated!

The upshot of all this is that the surgeon of today can best fulfil his objective – and his obligations – as a member of a team whose several and differing skills and judgments are mobilized at the earliest possible phase of this challenging disease. In none of the ills to which human flesh is heir is the wisdom of the many to be preferred to the decision, the wisdom or even the executive brilliance of the individual more than in cancer.

The rest of this chapter seeks to examine the surgical contribution to the cancer problem in respect to prevention, diagnosis and treatment. It is based on the sort of situations, and practices for which patients sometimes seek an explanation, and which the doctor sometimes fails to answer satisfactorily.

THE PLACE OF SURGERY IN CANCER PREVENTION

Certain conditions are now known to be precursors of cancer, and radical treatment of them will relieve the afflicted individual of this hazard.

Lumps in the thyroid gland in the neck, gallstones and familial warts in the lower bowel are in this category. Not all thyroid lumps carry the risk of cancer, of course, but there is no way of telling which do, and so the surgeon knows that for safety all should be removed.

Gallstones – a very common disease – may exist for a very long time without declaring their presence and may only be discovered casually, as by the radiologist when a person has to have an X-ray examination for some other cause – pain in the back, for example – or by the surgeon operating for some other abdominal complaint. Once discovered, it is wise policy to remove the gallbladder and the stones, unless the patient is too old or in too poor shape. The surgeon recommends this because he knows that, though 'silent' at the moment, gallstones can give rise to severe complications other than cancer, and that cancer in the gallbladder is never found in the absence of stones; and unhappily, when the growth is at length discovered, it is usually so far advanced as to be incurable.

In familial 'warts' of the bowel lining, an inherited disorder, a change to cancer is inevitable and early. The only safeguard is extensive removal of the affected bowel. For this reason members of families on the 'black list' are asked to undergo examination, and if they are afflicted they are advised – even in the absence of symptoms – to submit to operation. Usually an attempt is made to preserve the external aperture of the bowel even though its lining is not free from the disease. This is permissible only because this area is easy to examine, and an untoward change can be detected early. The patient, therefore, must remain under surveillance for the rest of his life.

Ulceration of the stomach is sometimes held to be precancerous. If this is ever so, the chances are so small that the risk of cancer should not weigh with the surgeon in deciding for or against surgery. On the other hand, it is not always possible to state categorically that an ulcer found by the radiologist is simple and operation may be the most certain way of finding out, though today our diagnostic resources are greatly increased. It is a good rule that a stomach ulcer that is not completely healed in three months should be operated upon.

In deciding for or against surgery in known malignant precursors, the surgeon has to balance the risk of operation and the possible mutilation against the risk of cancer supervening in the particular patient. In high risk situations – the familial warts of the colon, and certain forms of chronic ulceration of the bowel – there can be no doubt as to the wisdom of prophylactic surgery. Though operation has to be extensive, it offers complete protection, and at no other stage in these diseases can the assurance of complete cure be given.

THE ROLE OF SURGERY IN THE DIAGNOSIS OF CANCER

There is seldom any doubt about the diagnosis of established cancer, but in its early stages and in certain sites there may be no more than suspicion. In this event the surgeon has an important role. This may take one of two forms. The first is the detection of internal tumours when other methods of diagnosis have failed to come up with a positive answer, or when the disease has affected an organ or a part of an organ the clinical diagnostician is not yet able to investigate thoroughly. Operations to allow inspection of the internal organs are known as 'exploratory'. Fortunately they are required less and less often as investigative techniques become more and more sophisticated; but the risk of such exploratory operations is so infinitesimal that it should not be omitted. It is better to look and see than wait and see!

The second diagnostic procedure to which the surgeon can contribute is *biopsy*. This consists of the removal of tissue for microscopic study by the pathologist. When the tumour is small, it is generally removed in its entirety – an 'excision biopsy' – as in the case of a breast lump or a nodule in the thyroid. If the lesion is larger, or when the best mode of treatment may be in doubt, only a small portion is removed. Whenever possible the tissue removed is frozen, stained and submitted to immediate scrutiny by the pathologist, who more often than not is able at once to give an unequivocal diagnosis. In this event, the surgeon can proceed immediately with a definitive operation; but, so far as is known, a delay of a few days for more detailed pathological study is not harmful.

The tissue for biopsy may be obtained in various ways. The procedure may consist of nothing more than the withdrawal, through a needle inserted into the growth, of a small core of

137

tumour tissue; or of the removal of a small piece from the edge of a superficial ulcer, or of a portion of a projecting tumour by special forceps; or, in the case of tumours below the surface, by excising a portion through an incision in the skin. In the case of cancer of the womb the tissue is obtained by curettage, a minor operation in which the lining of the womb is gently scraped off.

In many instances the diagnosis is so obvious that biopsy is not required, but in some tumours it is quite imperative to obtain absolute confirmation before operation. This is particularly so when the radical treatment of a cancer will lead to mutilation, as for example when a limb tumour demands amputation, or the treatment of a cancer of the lower bowel may leave the patient with an opening on the front of the belly. No surgeon would dream of resorting to either of these irreversible procedures – or indeed to the removal of a breast – unless the diagnosis had been established beyond the shadow of a doubt.

The question of the possible harm a biopsy may do is often raised. It is impossible, of course, to deny that it may sometimes be harmful; on the other hand there is no good evidence that it is, provided the diagnosis is made promptly and is followed expeditiously by proper and definitive treatment.

ROLE OF SURGERY IN THE TREATMENT OF CANCER

The aims of the surgical treatment of cancer are twofold : firstly, 'curative', i.e. to eradicate the disease; or secondly, 'palliative', i.e. to relieve pain and distress, and maybe, to prolong life.

Few would disagree that the most satisfactory situation in the field of cancer therapy, is when a tumour is recognized early and the surgeon is able to remove it in its entirety. Unfortunately this is not always possible, and it then is desirable for a policy of management to be worked out by the surgeon in consultation with any colleagues whose particular skill may provide an acceptable alternative to surgery, or a complement or supplement to operation at the time or later.

'Curative' Surgery

The surgeon is sometimes asked if it is ever possible to cure cancer by operation. The query is prompted by the fact that everyone knows persons in whom operation has failed; the many successes are less publicized and are known only to close relatives and associates. The fact that the surgeon can cure cancer has been disputed, but mainly by statisticians, and by some who believe that the outcome of any individual cancer is uninfluenced by therapy and predetermined by the inherent nature of the tumour. This is an attitude of despair that no clinician can afford to countenance. The lie is given to it by the unquestioned progress in the last thirty to forty years in such common cancers as those of the breast, the bowel, and the mouth; though there are others in which our efforts have so far been less successful – the lung and the stomach, for example.

The belief that cancers are curable by operation rests on the concept that most begin as a localized change in the tissue, grow at varying rates in the original situation and then spread more widely, first to nearby glands, and then eventually by the blood to distant parts of the body. Every clinician knows of patients with tumours which have pursued a more unusual or bizarre course – some have even disappeared – but by and large the disease follows the pattern indicated. The corollary is that, caught in its early stages, it can be completely eradicated.

The essential feature of curative cancer surgery is that it should be adequate. To be so, the growth and its local surroundings must be cleanly and completely removed, with a safety margin of uninvolved normal tissue. The surgeon has to rely on his knowledge of the natural history of the disease and his experience to determine what constitutes the safety margin in this local part of the operation. It may entail the removal of a whole organ such as the breast or the thyroid gland, the stomach or the kidney; or it may demand the sacrifice of a limb, as in some forms of malignancy in bone, and some soft tissue tumours, even when quite small, such as the malignant mole. In certain forms of superficial cancer – as in the condition known as rodent ulcer – the margin of safety may be quite modest.

As a rule, the radical operation for curable cancer includes removal of the glands which are nearest the tumour and therefore the most likely to be involved when the disease spreads from its original site. This step is sometimes omitted, especially when there is no obvious disease in the glands; and sometimes the gland area is treated by irradiation, instead of surgery, or treatment

139

is postponed until evidence of involvement appears. Surgeons have not made up their minds absolutely on these respective policies. Some believe that the glands may constitute a defensive mechanism, as they are when enlarged in septic lesions, say, of the fingers. An answer to this may be forth-coming relatively soon, for the matter is under intensive study. In the meantime the evidence suggests that to delay an attack on the glands is not prejudicial to survival.

In superficial and observable cancers it is generally easy to select the potentially curable ones. In the case of internal tumours the decision for or against radical operation, and its scope, can be made only when the tumour is displayed at operation, and its possible ramifications investigated.

Unfortunately radical surgery may leave in its wake a legacy of considerable deformity, which at first sight is distressing, (and not least to the surgeon, who may indeed be deterred by compassion from offering it to the patient). Removal of the jaws, of the larynx, and high amputations at the shoulder and the hip are in this category. The surgeon must not be timid in urging the necessity for such ablations, or of discussing their merits and demerits; but the choice is ultimately the patient's own responsibility. In advising radical surgery it may be pointed out that there are ingenious devices – such as the artificial larynx and protheses both for arm and leg of increasing sophistication and efficiency – which help to minimize the disablement and disguise the deformity.

So far in the context of this chapter, surgery has meant operation by the use of the scalpel. Other means of ablation are now available, however. The electric current (or diathermy) has been in use for cutting, and for destroying small tumours for many years – a modern variant, perhaps, of the caustic unguents of long ago. Lately a new tool has been evolved in the shape of a cryogenic applicator which develops intense cold at its tip. 'Cryogenic surgery', as the new technique is called, has been used in the destruction of certain tumours of the brain, some superficial skin cancers and cancer of the prostate gland in men. The method is yet in its infancy, and time will have to elapse before its permanent value in the cancer surgeon's armamentarium can be determined.

The safety of modern surgery has posed some difficult problems

140

for the surgeon. Appreciating – and believing – that early cancer is curable, should he opt for extensive local procedures – 'wide excision' – in order to make sure? Should he resort in early disease to the sort of operation usually reserved for more advanced cancers – as, for example, to remove the entire stomach in early gastric cancer? Should he, in fact, carry out larger and larger operations for smaller and smaller tumours. Most would be deterred from so doing if the bigger operation meant mutilation or greater disablement, but equally most would feel impelled to do so if there was – or when there is – proof that such a policy offered a substantially better chance of complete cure.

It is this kind of outlook that has stimulated some surgeons to design primary operations which might be called 'super radical', and others to regard reappearance of the disease after orthodox primary removal as a challenge to be met by even more heroic attempts at extensive ablation. There is no great scope for this sort of surgery, perhaps; but it must be conceded to have an occasional place in the curative repertoire of surgery. It is wrong to reject the concept of 'super radical' surgery through ignorance of its possibilities, or repugnance to practise it. It demands of the surgeon courage, possibly humane ruthlessness, and certainly technical virtuosity of a high order. Its most important practical application is when disease has extended from its original site to involve organs and tissues in its immediate vicinity without yet having spread to more distant areas.

ROLE OF SURGERY IN THE PALLIATION OF CANCER

When cancer has advanced to a stage at which cure is impossible, or the disease is irremovable, or when it has recurred, further treatment is 'palliative'. This implies that it is intended to relieve, as far as possible, the distressing and disabling *sequelae* of the disease. In this humane exercise surgery has often an important part to play, sometimes alone, sometimes in concert with irradiation, hormone treatment, or the use of anti-cancer drugs.

There was a time when advanced or recurrent cancer was a signal for 'throwing in the sponge', and confining any therapy to making 'less rugged the inevitable pathway to the tomb'.

A different philosophy governs the attitude of the surgeon of today—a reluctance to acknowledge defeat, a desire to prolong life, and to control and abate for as long as possible the worst and most incapacitating manifestations of the disease.

There is no doubt that life may be usefully prolonged by surgery, and without discomfort even when eradication of the disease is impracticable. This is so in such cancers as those of the gullet, the stomach and the bowel, which may cause fatal mechanical obstruction long before the disease is strictly terminal. Palliative removal of such tumours not only prevents such complications as death by starvation or obstruction, but may add materially to the comfort of the patient. Apart from this there is some evidence that even when fatal mechanical complications are unlikely removal of the main bulk of a tumour may allow the natural defensive mechanisms of the body to hold off, at least for a time, the activities of the remaining malignant tissues.

The prolongation of life is not the main yardstick of palliative therapeutics, however; few would choose to live longer in order to suffer more; and a more important aspect of palliation is the relief it may afford of the more distressing *sequelae* of incurable cancer. Thus operation is the surest and quickest way of getting rid of a foul, ulcerating infected or bleeding mass of malignant tissue, both on the surface of the body and in some internal situations. It is the only way of bypassing abnormal penetrations of a cancer into another organ. These are two of the more depressing *sequelae* of advanced cancer, for both make the patient repugnant to himself and, unfortunately, to others, so that their alleviation is a considerable social as well as therapeutic achievement.

There are other forms of palliative surgery—the short circuit of a growth causing jaundice or of one causing bowel or bladder difficulties, for example—but three other ameliorating treatment policies have considerable contemporary importance :

1. Some tumours spread to the skeleton, and by destroying the substance of the bone lead to fractures. Such lesions are known as 'pathological' fractures; and though at one time they often doomed the patient to become bed-ridden, the modern orthopaedic surgeon is often able to remove the disease and insert a metallic or plastic substitute for the affected part of the bone.

2. The discovery that the behaviour of some tumours can

be influenced by removing certain of the glands — endocrine glands — that normally control many of the body's activities has been exploited in some forms of widely disseminated cancer originating in organs known to be subject to such control — the breast, the thyroid gland, and the prostate, for example. In a proportion of patients, treatment by the administration of the products of the controlling glands, or removal or destruction of the glands themselves, may bring about a considerable degree of relief (see Chapter IX).

3.   The pain of advanced cancer is probably its greatest and most wearing tribulation. Unfortunately some cancers induce pain some time before they normally cause death, and in such an event the early resort to pain-killing drugs is distasteful, or resented both by patient and relatives. The neurological surgeon has much to offer in this situation, by destructive injections into the nerves carrying the impulses of pain, or by comparatively minor operations on the pain pathways in the spinal cord or the brain itself.

The author of this chapter is a surgeon who has tried to indicate the place of surgery in the present day management of cancer. It should not be assumed that he — or any other surgeon — is satisfied with this contribution, gratifying though some parts of it are. The future lies elsewhere than in the operating room; but when the answer is eventually found, the surgeon will have no cause to be ashamed of his attempts to relieve suffering and not infrequently avert the arrows of death in one of the greatest scourges of mankind.

CHAPTER VII

RADIOTHERAPY

ERIC EASSON

This chapter is concerned with radiotherapy, what it means, how it works, the conditions for which it is useful, and in particular what kind of response can be expected with certain kinds of cancer.

THE EVOLUTION OF RADIOTHERAPY

The branch of Medicine known as Therapeutics is concerned with the treatment of disease by various agencies, chemical, physical, psychological. Radiotherapy or radiation therapeutics is one aspect of the general field of therapeutics and is concerned with the treatment of disease, mainly malignant disease, by certain penetrating radiations. The relevant radiations are known collectively as ionising radiations because one of the effects they create on passing through matter of any kind (including gases) is to split off electrons from their parent atoms, thus producing highly reactive ions. It is interesting to see how these therapeutically-useful radiations are related to other well-known types of radiant energy such as radio waves and the several components of visible light. Figure 37 shows the so-called electro-magnetic spectrum, ranging from the relatively long radio waves through the visible spectrum to X-rays and gamma rays.

Cancer is as old as life itself, but it was not until 1895 that Roëntgen discovered X-rays, while in 1896 Becquerel discovered the radio-activity in uranium. Pierre and Marie Curie then isolated radium and the other radio-active constituents of uranium. Within ten years X-rays were being commonly used to display broken bones and other abnormalities, and diagnostic radiology was born. Also within a decade of their discovery, X-rays and the gamma rays from radium were found to have profound biological effects, the most important of which was their

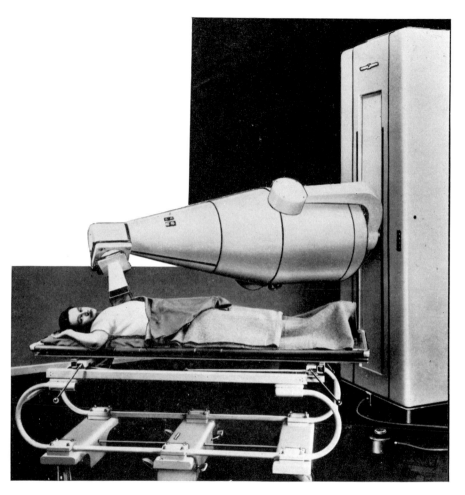

PLATE I: Conventional X-ray machine producing X-rays with an energy of 300,000 volts.

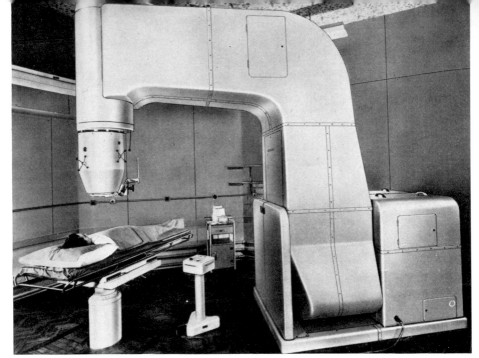

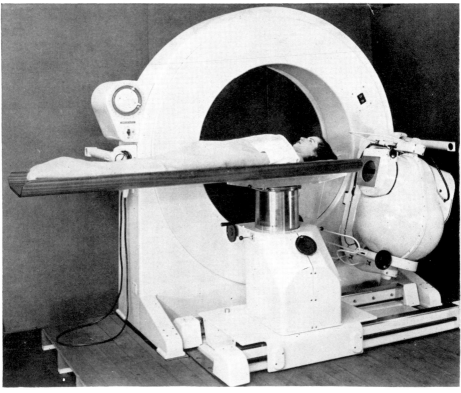

PLATE II: Above, Linear accelerator machine producing X-rays with an energy of 4 million volts, *below*, telecobalt machine producing gamma rays with an energy equivalent to 3 million volt X-rays.

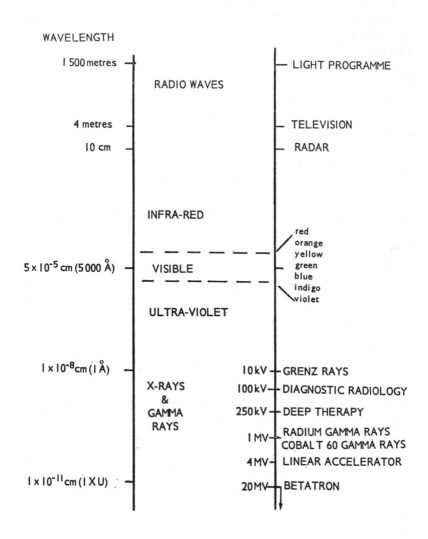

WAVELENGTH

1 500 metres — — LIGHT PROGRAMME

RADIO WAVES

4 metres — — TELEVISION

10 cm — — RADAR

INFRA-RED

red
orange
yellow
5×10^{-5} cm (5 000 Å) — VISIBLE — green
blue
indigo
violet

ULTRA-VIOLET

1×10^{-8} cm (1 Å) — 10 kV — GRENZ RAYS

X-RAYS 100 kV — DIAGNOSTIC RADIOLOGY
&
GAMMA 250 kV — DEEP THERAPY
RAYS
1 MV — RADIUM GAMMA RAYS
COBALT 60 GAMMA RAYS

4 MV — LINEAR ACCELERATOR

1×10^{-11} cm (1 XU) — 20 MV — BETATRON

FIGURE 37

Diagram of electro-magnetic spectrum showing the relative energies of different radiations including those employed in radiotherapy. Å represents Angstram units [1Å = 10^{-8} cm.]

inhibiting effect on malignant growths and indeed on any growing or active tissue such as normal blood-forming marrow. Thus, by 1910, radiotherapy too had been born – though great developments lay ahead.

In the early days the rather primitive X-ray tubes were in fact employed for both diagnostic and therapeutic purposes, and by the same workers : radium on the other hand, since it was normally inserted into tissues and body cavities under general anaesthesia, was employed by surgeons and gynaecologists. It was not until the 1930s that radiotherapy began to make rapid progress as a special discipline, when a small number of far-sighted enthusiasts, aided by equally enthusiastic physicists, realized that the biological effects of X-rays and of gamma rays were qualitatively similar and should be explored and developed together. Great improvements in the design of X-ray tubes assisted this development, but of special importance was the recognition of the need for accurate and reliable measurement of dosage. As with other therapeutic agents, where a dose of a drug must be precisely measured in terms of milligrams, and administered in a carefully planned sequence of doses over a predetermined period, so also with radiotherapy, for which small groups of devoted radiation physicists developed a precise dosage unit appropriately called the roentgen unit. It was then possible to determine, with clinical consistency, how much ionising radiation was necessary, in a given overall time, to create the desired biological effects. Moreover, proper procedures were established and agreed internationally, for the safe handling and maintenance of all sources of therapeutic (and diagnostic) radiations. Thus 'modern' radiotherapy became established, the new discipline was soundly based on physical principles, made safe for both patients and staff, and well prepared for the great advances in nuclear physics which the atomic pile and the atomic bomb were to make possible. Shortly after the end of World War II, large quantities of 'artificial' radioactive substances (isotopes) became available from nuclear reactors and the naturally occurring radium became only one of a wide range of weapons in the radiotherapist's armamentarium. Many of these artificial radioactive isotopes are employed as radium-substitutes, each with its own unique characteristics of special value to the radiotherapist under appropriate circumstances. For example, the metal cobalt can be made intensely radioactive, in small bulk, and housed in a protective block of steel in such a way as to emit a controllable beam of gamma rays with a penetrating power equivalent to X-rays generated at about 3 million volts. These telecobalt machines have proved of immense value throughout the world. At the same time multi-million volt or 'megavoltage' X-ray machines were being developed, based on entirely new physical principles, and capable of producing X-rays of great penetrating power. Whereas machines of the late 1930s and 1940s produced X-rays with an energy of 250,000 volts, the new machines, linear accelerators and betatrons, were now producing X-ray energies ranging from 3 or 4 to 30 or more million volts. Thus, where the gamma rays of radium were once regarded as the most penetrating of known radiations, with an energy-equivalent of about 1 million volts, X-rays were now available which greatly exceeded this energy. The new X-ray and telecobalt machines also provided many other technical advantages which *in toto* very greatly simplified and improved the radiotherapeutic management of patients with cancer.

The radiotherapy department of today has a range of machines each providing X-rays of different energy and suitable for specific clinical purposes. Superficial cancers, affecting for example the skin, require X-rays with not too great a penetrating power, and for such purposes an energy of from 60 to 100 kilovolts is employed. For more deeply seated cancers X-rays are used with an energy of from 300 kilovolts to 4 or 10 million volts–or even higher (Plates I and II). Some X-ray machines (linear accelerators and betatrons) can also be used to produce a beam of electrons, and these have some special advantages in selected cases because of their limited and controllable penetrating power. Electrons can, for example, be used to irradiate a superficial plaque of tissue without penetrating more deeply, thus sparing the underlying normal tissues. More recently beams of neutrons have become available and their unique features will be discussed later when future prospects are considered.

In addition to X-ray or 'beam' machines, the radiotherapy department has a range of radioactive isotopes. Radium, a naturally occurring isotope, is still of considerable importance and is used in the form of 'needles' and tubes of differing dimensions. Various artificial isotopes are also employed as 'radium substitutes'–radioactive cobalt, caesium, gold, yttrium, iridium, tantalum, and others–all with their own unique physical and biological characteristics on which their therapeutic usefulness depends. Like radium these substances may be implanted into the tissues in the form of seeds or 'needles', inserted into body cavities such as the womb, or may be applied in close contact with the skin to irradiate a superficial plaque of tumour. Apart from the 'solid' radioactive isotopes certain isotopes in solution have their therapeutic place, notably radioactive iodine, phosphorus, and colloidal gold.

The effective and safe use of all these sources of therapeutic radiation demands not only trained medical specialists (radio-therapists) but much additional team work. The physicist is a vital member of this team, and it is he and his technicians who ensure that all the machines are working properly and that the radiation doses prescribed by the doctor do actually reach the patient's tumour. A special department, known as a Mould Room, is concerned with the preparation of plastic 'shells' and 'moulds', each made to measure for individual patients, and providing a high-precision jig by which each carefully measured beam of X-rays hits the bull's eye (the centre of the tumour) each and every time the patient is treated. Highly qualified technicians prepare these 'beam-direction' shells, and equally highly trained radiographers carry out the daily treatments. The technical skill of the latter is combined with a knowledge of nursing and general patient care–so necessary in creating a sense of confidence in the anxious patient.

Emphasis has been put on the importance of precision in directing therapeutic radiations to the right place in the right quantity and at the right time. Clearly this technical precision is to the radiotherapist what operative skill and dexterity are to the surgeon. However, such technical skills, while essential to success, must be combined with medical experience and sound clinical judgment–no less in the radiotherapist than in the surgeon.

BIOLOGICAL EFFECTS

How do these therapeutic radiations work? What therapeutically useful biological effects do they create? At one time, early in this century, the answers to these questions seemed fairly simple and straightforward; but, like so many aspects of modern science, complexity leads to even greater complexity, and the discipline of radiobiology now attracts thousands of scientists seeking to elucidate the subtle changes induced by the passage of ionising radiations through tissues. The radiation chemist explores, detects and measures the infinitely tiny and momentary chemical changes created by ionising radiations. From his studies, too, came the first prospects of radiation-protecting and -sensitizing substances. The geneticist studies the effects of radiations on genes and chromosomes, mapping the subtle changes reflected in the adult animal. Cellular and tissue-culture studies lead on to the effects of radiation on whole animals. All these effects are correlated with known effects in man observed during and after necessary treatment of his cancers.

In brief, ionising radiations have the capacity to damage all living cells, whether cancerous or not. The greatest effect of these radiations is seen in the nucleus of a cell, and especially so when the nucleus and its surrounding cytoplasm are about to divide to make two cells – the process of mitosis. Cells can be shown to have somewhat different degrees of vulnerability to radiations, depending on the phase of the mitotic cycle during which they are irradiated. The degree of damage to a cell depends also, and principally, on the quantity or dose of radiation given to the cell. The amount of damage to a culture of cells, or to a 'tissue of cells' is expressed in terms of their capacity to continue reproducing themselves. So far as a cancerous cell is concerned the object of irradiation is to damage the cell so that it cannot reproduce itself again and will instead degenerate and die. An associated object of such treatment is to give the malignant tumour such a measured dosage of X- or gamma rays that the cancer cells will stop reproducing but the normal body cells in which the tumour lies will not be damaged beyond their powers of recovery and they will retain their normal function and reproductive capacity.

Ionising radiations are known to alter the chemical constitution and consequently the biochemical function, of, for example, cellular enzymes – those vital substances so essential to the control of the body's total chemistry, at all levels from complex tissues to intra-cellular and even intra-nuclear activities. These

149

radiations can also disrupt chromosomes in many different ways, the breakages and abnormal linkages being readily visible microscopically. Physical or physico-chemical damage to individual genes can also be demonstrated by suitable genetic studies.

At a more visible level of observation, X- and gamma rays create an intense inflammatory reaction in human and animal tissues. The intensity and duration of this inflammatory reaction depends primarily on the dosage of radiation given. One of the first effects of X-rays to be noted by early workers in this field was the inhibition of bone-marrow activity. This is reflected in the blood as a fall in the number of circulating white blood cells, and once more the extent of this effect, and its duration, are directly related to dosage – a small dose of X-rays may result in no measurable effect on the blood, a much larger dose could result in total marrow failure and death – as with the victims of the atom bombs in Hiroshima and Nagasaki at the end of World War II. Exploiting this effect on blood-forming tissue, one of the earliest therapeutic applications of X-rays (about 1902) was in the treatment of leukaemia. (This method of treatment is still employed, though chemotherapy has some advantages in chronic leukaemia and is the treatment of choice in acute leukaemia.) Malignant tumours being characterized by cell multiplication ionising radiations likewise inhibit such growths. When, and how best to achieve permanent inhibition of malignant growths is the province of radiotherapy.

CLINICAL ASPECTS

How are these biological effects applied at a clinical level in man? Though the indications for its use are limited in number, radiotherapy does have a great deal to offer in the management of certain non-malignant or benign diseases. For example, a small dose of X-rays directed at the ovaries can, by inhibiting further development of egg cells, stop menstrual bleeding, and can therefore be of immense value to those women who are sometimes plagued by heavy and often unpredictable bleeding when they reach the age of the menopause. For those patients suffering from excessive activity of the thyroid gland (causing loss of weight, sweating, palpitation of the heart and a rapid pulse, tremulousness and muscle weakness, prominent eyes, and often

150

enlargement of the thyroid gland) a simple tasteless drink of radioactive iodine provides an elegant and, of course, non-surgical method of treatment, and a rapid return to normal health. Since the thyroid gland cannot biochemically distinguish a radioactive from a non-radioactive atom of iodine, it absorbs these atoms into its functioning cells which are then irradiated and killed from within–by millions of atomic Trojan horses! The perceptive reader will promptly ask if cancer of the thyroid gland can be similarly attacked. The answer is that it certainly can–but alas, only rarely to any significant extent. Unhappily, malignant tumours of the thyroid–or indeed any other organ–are so busy growing, their cancerous cells dividing to such an extent, that they cannot settle down to perform their normal function of absorbing iodine and synthesizing the normal secretion of that gland. In short, cells cannot both multiply and function at the same time. This is indeed one of the greatest disappointments in post-war cancer therapy. (Thyroid cancer can in fact respond to external X-ray therapy, usually after preliminary surgical excision.)

Fortunately there are many forms of cancer for which other radiotherapeutic measures can be highly effective, and in suitable circumstances truly curative. Early experience demonstrated that malignant tumours differ widely in their responsiveness to irradiation. Some tumours are quite resistant to irradiation at tolerable levels of dosage, while at the other end of the scale there are types of cancer which disappear completely and permanently in response to relatively low dosage. Why there should be such wide differences in response is one of the fields of interest to radiobiologists, and a great deal of research effort is being directed to the elucidation of this problem. To the clinical radiotherapist the fact remains that, for example, cancer of the stomach or of the colon is not a rewarding type of cancer to treat by this method (the treatment of choice being surgical). Some 'radio-resistant' tumours can actually continue to enlarge visibly in spite of vigorous irradiation. On the other hand, cancer of the mouth and throat, of the skin, the bladder, and the uterine cervix, show very gratifying results. Certain other types of cancer affecting lymphatic glands, such as Hodgkin's disease (and a number of variants of that disease) are exceedingly 'sensitive' to X-rays. The term radio-sensitivity in this context refers to the relative rate of response and the diminution in size of the tumour following irradiation. For reasons which we shall not discuss here (and which are largely unknown in any case) radio-sensitivity and curability are not synonymous terms. In fact, most of the cancers cured by radiotherapy are only moderately sensitive, though some of the most highly curable are indeed also highly sensitive.

Everyone appreciates that a surgical operation is attended by discomfort, sometimes acute and even prolonged, but this is tolerated as the acceptable price of success. Radiotherapy likewise may be associated with a period of discomfort which must be accepted in the interests of curing the patient of his cancer. The inflammatory nature of a radiation reaction has already been mentioned, and during a course of treatment a patient may in some circumstances develop an 'inflamed' throat (discomfort on swallowing) or an inflamed bladder (frequent passing of scalding urine) or bowel (diarrhoea) – depending on the organ or tissue irradiated. These transient symptoms can be alleviated to a large extent by suitable medicine and in truth are no more troublesome than the post-operative upset so readily accepted by surgical patients. Radiotherapy patients may also be helped simply by explaining away the mystique of these invisible 'rays', for some so-called radiation sickness is undoubtedly psychogenic and based on fear of the unknown.

A period of temporary morbidity therefore is an acceptable consequence of radiotherapy when the object of the treatment is permanent cure of a cancer. There are many occasions, however, when a patient may have a tumour which is too extensive for surgical removal, and too large for curative irradiation. Nevertheless, for such patients radiotherapy can often provide considerable relief of symptoms, e.g. relief of pain, healing of a pathological fracture, healing of a discharging ulcer, and sometimes substantial prolongation of a useful life. When such palliation is the therapeutic object prolonged periods of treatment in hospital are avoided, and so also are the more tiresome side effects of treatment.

There are some cancers for which surgical excision (if technically feasible) is undoubtedly the treatment of choice, e.g. for cancer of the rectum. On the other hand there are cancers for which radiotherapy is the proper line of treatment –

for example, tumours of the lymphatic system. There are a number of cancers – such as cancer of the larynx, of the mouth, and of the uterine cervix – for which radiotherapy is usually preferred to surgery because the latter would involve considerable loss of function as, for example, the loss of normal speech if the larynx is removed. In such cases radiotherapy is the first line of attack, with surgical excision kept in reserve only for those patients for whom radiotherapy fails to cure. Finally, there are the cancers which are best managed by a judicious combination of surgery and radiotherapy, for example, when the surgeon opens the bladder and removes all but the base of a projecting tumour, while the radiotherapist inserts radioactive gold grains to kill off any cancer cells left in the bladder wall. Thus the radiotherapist and a variety of surgeons – general, ear-nose-and-throat, urological, neurosurgical, thoracic, and plastic surgeons – all work in close harmony in order to provide the best possible chance for cure.

Radiotherapy and surgery may also be combined, where necessary, with chemotherapy, i.e. with various cytotoxic drugs. These are discussed in detail in the next chapter.

How effective can radiotherapy be in the treatment of cancer? Plates III and IV show two typical and easily demonstrable examples of cancers responding to irradiation. It must be emphasized again, however, that the curability of any cancer depends primarily on its dimensions at the time of treatment. A very large mass of cancer is unlikely to respond permanently to radiotherapy, and of course, even a small primary is incurable by available therapy, if the tumour has already shed secondary deposits via the blood stream to more remote parts of the body. Nevertheless, it is important to appreciate that substantial numbers of patients with various types of cancers are amenable to permanent cure provided the circumstances are right – and it is important to try to ensure that more and more patients are treated under these favourable conditions, so far as this lies within our control.

For several decades it has been customary to express the effectiveness of cancer treatment in terms of five-year survival-rates, i.e. the percentage of patients who are alive five years after appropriate treatment. This arbitrary five-year interval has provided a useful yardstick to evaluate the different methods of treatment within any one centre, and also between many different centres throughout the world. It is instructive, however, to look at this matter in terms of definitive cure, and this can be precisely defined as follows. We can speak of cure of cancer when there remains a group of disease-free survivors, at intervals of from five to ten or more years after treatment, whose annual death rate from all causes is identical to that of a normal population of the same sex and age distribution. This is not only a statistically-valid definition of cure but it is of course a very reassuring one for the cancer patient. It also provides great encouragement for the cancer therapist, for he can now see that many of his patients can be given a perfectly normal expectation of life. Studies of curability along the lines mentioned above have also disclosed that some cancers, e.g. Hodgkin's disease, which were once deemed incurable, can indeed enjoy a normal life-expectancy after appropriate treatment under favourable conditions. The need now is to try to achieve similar results in higher proportions of all cancer patients.

THE FUTURE

What does the future hold? What further improvements in the effectiveness of radiation therapy can be expected? With modern machines the radiotherapist can now select a variety of beams of X-rays with ingenious modifying filters designed to irradiate a malignant tumour in any part of the body, and of any shape or size. Techniques are now carefully planned to confine the radiation almost entirely to the tumour itself, sparing the normal tissues in a way that could formerly only be done by implanted radium – and even then in only a few selected and accessible sites. From a purely technical point of view therefore it is difficult to imagine any significant improvement in the process of delivering a required dose of X-rays to any tumour.

From a biological point of view, however, a number of interesting possibilities are being actively investigated. For example, certain chemical agents are known to protect living cells from the effects of irradiation, and it would be clearly advantageous if normal tissues could be protected in such a way that higher and more effective dosage could be directed at the tumour. Unfortunately the available protective agents are either unpleasantly toxic in man or, almost worse, they not only protect normal tissues but they protect the tumour as well. An alternative approach to this problem is to devise some means of increasing the sensitivity of cells to the effects of irradiation and this at the moment does hold some promise. Once again, however, what is required is some means of increasing the radio-sensitivity of the tumour without at the same time increasing the sensitivity and vulnerability of the normal tissues in and around the tumour. Some ten or fifteen years ago it was observed that living cells were much more vulnerable to the effects of irradiation if they were artificially maintained at a high level of oxygenation. *Per contra*, they were also found to be resistant to the effects of irradiation if they were irradiated under anoxic conditions. Moreover, it seems probable that certain tumours fail to resolve permanently after irradiation because some of their cells contain little oxygen and are consequently less vulnerable to ionising radiation. These cells may later multiply to produce a substantial and lethal tumour. These radiobiological findings have led to three possibilities at a clinical level :

1. It is possible, but clearly unacceptable, to render a whole patient anoxic or even hypoxic by some artificial means because the brain cannot tolerate even short periods of reduced oxygen content. Nevertheless with some tumours occurring in the limbs it is possible by the application of a tourniquet to render the limb and the tumour within it relatively anoxic. Under such circumstances it has been found possible to deliver much higher doses of radiation than would have been tolerated under normal conditions. What has yet to be proved, however, is that such tumours become more curable, that is to say that a larger percentage of such patients are cured of their cancers, than would otherwise have been the case under conditions of normal oxygenation.

2. Efforts in the opposite direction have been made in many centres, by placing patients within a sealed chamber and increasing the atmospheric pressure within it. This 'hyperbaric oxygenation' has been shown, in experimental biological systems, to improve the oxygen content in the radio-resistant pockets of cells. It has also been shown that under hyperbaric conditions the patient's normal tissues and tumour are both undoubtedly

more sensitive to the effects of radiation, but once again it still remains to be proved that larger numbers of patients can have their cancers cured as a result of these treatment methods. This is a matter for continuing and carefully assessed studies and the results of these are awaited with great interest.

3. A third possibility, exploiting this same question of radio-resistance of hypoxic tumour cells, lies in the use of fast neutrons. It has been known for some ten or more years that fast neutrons, unlike X- and gamma rays, are less dependent for their effectiveness on the presence of oxygen in the tissues or tumour cells. Though formerly produced only by massive cyclotrons, beams of neutrons are now available from machines of modest and practical dimensions, and extensive clinical trials are anticipated within the next year or two. This is likely to prove one of the most interesting and exciting research projects in radiotherapy during the next decade.

CHAPTER VIII

CHEMOTHERAPY

T. CONNORS

Many of the diseases from which man suffers are the result of infection by various parasites including insects, worms, single cell organisms, bacteria, fungi and viruses. The eradication of these infections by specific treatment with chemicals is termed chemotherapy. A successful chemotherapeutic agent will be a chemical which is not poisonous to man but extremely toxic to the infecting organism. The agent will have no ill effects on man when taken but it will be distributed throughout the body, coming into contact with the parasites and killing them or preventing them from multiplying.

The treatment of parasitic infections by chemicals and mixtures of chemicals has been practised with varying degrees of success for many hundreds of years. As early as the seventeenth century moderately effective remedies were available for the treatment of such conditions as malaria (extract of cinchona bark was often effective) and amoebic dysentery (ipecacuanha root often controlled the more distressing symptoms of this infection).

Chemotherapy as a modern science began early in this century. Scientists infected rats and mice with parasites related to those found in man and measured the ability of chemicals to control the disease. In this way large numbers of chemicals could be 'screened' for their usefulness in combating a parasitic infection related to one occurring in man. Chemical compounds found to be active in these screening tests often proved to be successful when employed against the similar disease in man. In the past fifty years great progress has been made in the treatment of many infections, the most notable, of course, being the use of penicillin and other antibiotics in the treatment of diseases caused by bacteria. In other cases, however, particularly for virus diseases, effective chemotherapeutic agents have yet to be discovered.

CANCER CHEMOTHERAPY

In some ways cancer resembles a parasitic disease. Although not infectious, cancer cells live off the host in which they arise. Like many parasites they invade and destroy the normal tissues of the body and many cancers may similarly release toxic substances into the blood-stream. However, in two important ways cancer is quite dissimilar from any parasitic infection.

1. Invading parasites are recognized as foreign by the body and man's immunological mechanisms attempt to reject these organisms in the same way, for example, as a transplanted kidney is recognized as foreign and rejected (unless measures are taken to eliminate these immunological defences). A parasitic infection may eventually overwhelm man but it does so only in the face of a continuous challenge from the body's natural defences. Cancer cells, unfortunately, are not recognized as foreign by the body in the same way and the body's attempts to reject them are either very weak, or non-existent. The treatment of cancer by chemicals can, therefore, be seen to be a much more difficult proposition than the treatment of parasitic disease. In the latter case the administered chemical will only have to kill a proportion of the invading organisms and leave the rest to be destroyed by the body's immune response. In the former case the chemical may be required to kill every single cancer cell.

2. A chemotherapeutic agent must be toxic to the invading parasite but well tolerated by the host. It is easy to understand how a chemical can be harmless to man but poisonous to an organism far removed in structure and metabolism. Penicillin, for instance, kills bacteria because it interferes with the formation of their cell wall. It is quite harmless to man because the walls of human cells are quite different in their composition and structure. But cancer cells have arisen from normal cells and retain much of their original identity. Here the normal cell which must not be harmed by the chemical and the cancer cell which must be killed by the same chemical are very similar. As might be expected in such a situation chemicals which are found to be toxic to cancer cells are frequently just as toxic to man himself and not practicable as a form of treatment.

THE ROLE OF CHEMOTHERAPY

These features of cancer mean that it is difficult to find chemicals with the right properties for use in the treatment of cancer in man. Nevertheless the search for potential anti-cancer agents is carried out intensively all over the world because, for some cancers, chemotherapy is at present the only feasible form of treatment.

When the cancer is localized and has only invaded surrounding tissues to a limited extent it can, in many cases, be removed by surgery or completely destroyed by X-rays. Paradoxically, although cancer is a highly lethal disease it rarely gives early warning symptoms of its presence. Unless it arises in some obvious site such as skin, its presence may remain undetected until it is well advanced. Once a cancer has widely invaded surrounding tissues and spread throughout the body to form secondary cancers, surgery obviously becomes impracticable. Also much of the value of X-ray therapy, which can be very effective if it can be accurately focused on a tumour, is lost. In such cases chemotherapy is the only available form of treatment.

Tumours of the white blood cells, the leukaemias, are widely spread throughout the body when first diagnosed. The only treatment for these relatively common cancers is chemotherapy, and for this reason much of the attention of the research scientist is devoted to finding chemicals likely to be useful in the treatment of the various leukaemias.

The ultimate aim of chemotherapy is to achieve a complete cure and as with surgery and X-rays, it has the best chance of doing this if the cancer is treated at an early stage. On many occasions, chemotherapy is given as a last resort if surgery or radiotherapy have failed to halt the growth of the cancer. Under these conditions, chemotherapy may have slight effects and alleviate some of the symptoms of the disease (palliative chemotherapy) but it can rarely achieve a cure.

In the case of two quite rare cancers, choriocarcinoma and Burkitt's lymphoma, chemotherapy is given before either surgery or radiotherapy, and with a good expectancy of obtaining cures. The case of Burkitt's lymphoma is an interesting example of the progress of chemotherapy in recent years. This tumour, first described in detail by the surgeon, Mr Burkitt, only ten years

159

ago, is particularly prevalent in young children in certain parts of Africa. Because of poor medical facilities in the area, children were often taken for treatment at a time when the tumour was well advanced. Even when surgery was feasible at this late stage, there was a high mortality associated with the operation. Radiotherapy was not available in these regions and chemotherapy was given as the only available treatment. In many cases, as illustrated in Plate Va, the results were quite dramatic. Administration of chemicals which had been available for a number of years, caused complete regression of the tumour. In some cases the tumours have not reappeared for four years or more and the patients are considered cured. There is every hope that by studying this tumour further, one may be able to obtain complete cures in every instance.

Choriocarcinoma is a cancer of the placental tissues and less than twenty years ago it was an incurable disease. Today more than 80 per cent of patients with this cancer who are treated by chemotherapy are cured. Although quite a rare disease in England, this cancer is prevalent in some parts of the world and its eradication by chemotherapy represents one of the great contributions of chemotherapy to the treatment of cancer.

Chemotherapy also plays a role in combination with surgery or radiotherapy in the treatment of certain types of cancer. Chemicals may be given to reduce some tumours to a size at which they may be successfully treated by X-rays. In the treatment of some cancers, radiotherapy and chemicals given simultaneously or one immediately following the other, can have anti-tumour effects which could not be obtained by either treatment alone. After surgery, anti-cancer agents are sometimes given to destroy any tumour cells that may have escaped detection.

THE DETECTION OF ANTI-CANCER AGENTS BY SCREENING TESTS

The search for anti-cancer agents is conducted along similar lines to those used in the search for other types of chemotherapeutic agent. Chemicals are tested against animal models which simulate the disease in man. Obviously, to detect anti-cancer agents, one measures the effects of drugs in laboratory animals with cancer.

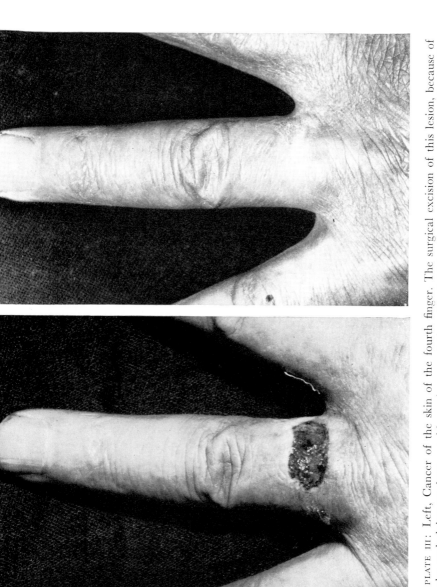

PLATE III: Left, Cancer of the skin of the fourth finger. The surgical excision of this lesion, because of the underlying tendons, would require amputation. The initial treatment of choice therefore is by irradiation, right. Photograph taken several years after treatment showing excellent result with normal function of the finger.

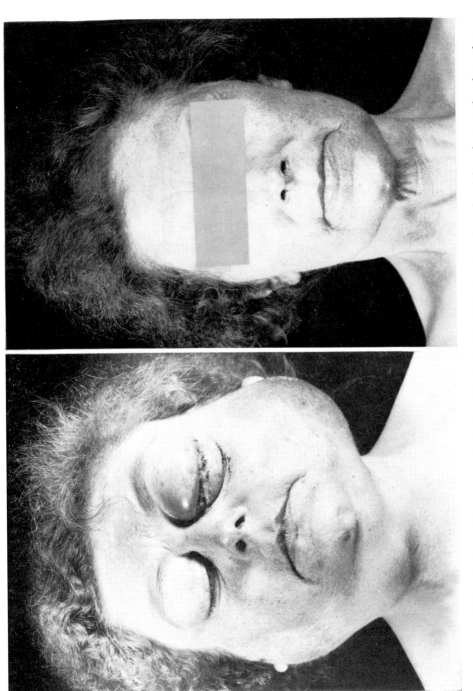

PLATE IV: *Left*, A substantial tumour of the lymphatic glands of the head and neck, *right*, photograph taken after treatment showing rapid and complete resolution.

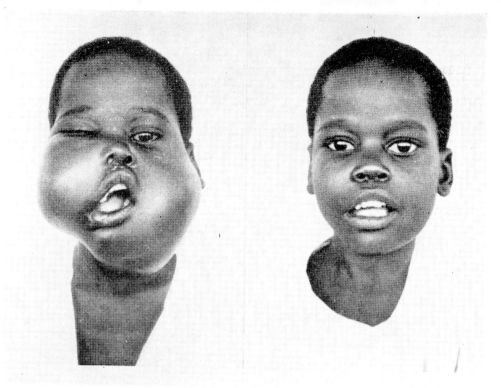

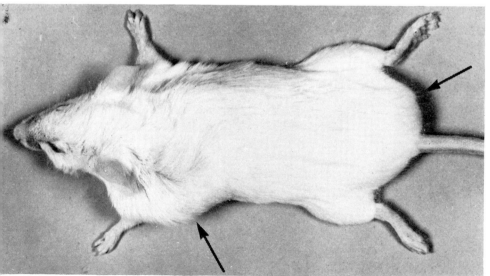

PLATE V:

Above, THE EFFECT OF CHEMOTHERAPY ON BURKITT'S LYMPHOMA
A single injection of a chemical causes a rapid reduction in size of the tumour. A fortnight after treatment the tumour has disappeared completely. In a number of cases the tumours had not regrown after four years or more. [P. Clifford, *East African Medical Journal, 1966*]

Below, A MOUSE WITH TWO MAMMARY TUMOURS
This mouse is of an inbred strain that has a very high incidence of these tumours.

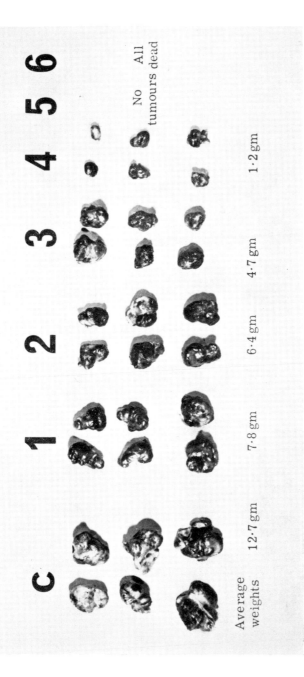

PLATE VI: SCREENING TEST ON A TRANSPLANTABLE TUMOUR

The tumours have been removed from rats one week after the test drug was administered. Small doses of the drug (Groups 1, 2) had not affected the tumour size which was similar in these groups to the control group (C). Group's 3, 4 tumours had been affected by the drug at higher doses while the dose given to Group 5 had cured the animals. The highest dose of all, given to Group 6, has killed all the animals.

Over the years several strains of rat and mouse have been obtained by continual in-breeding, and certain of these strains are prone to develop a high incidence of a particular cancer. Plate Vb shows a mouse with two breast cancers, from a strain that shows a very high incidence of these tumours. In this case, the cancer is caused by a virus which is transmitted from generation to generation in the milk of the mother.

Alternatively, cancers can be made to arise in animals by a number of methods such as the application of chemicals or the administration of viruses as described in earlier chapters. However, the most favoured method because it requires less space and a smaller number of animals is to obtain the tumours by transplantation. If a tumour arises in a rat or mouse either spontaneously or by chemical induction, it can often be transferred to rats or mice of a similar genetic character by means of small fragments of the tumour. Each fragment quickly grows to form another tumour which may similarly be transferred to more animals. In this way one tumour may be used to give rise to a large number of similar tumours, and it may be maintained for generation after generation.

TESTS USING TRANSPLANTED TUMOURS

In testing a new drug on a tumour-bearing animal the scientist attempts to answer two questions: (1) Can the drug affect the growth of the tumour or preferably cause it to disappear? (2) If the drug is effective what is the difference in the amount of drug that causes this effect and the amount of drug that kills the animal? To discover a chemical that causes a cancer to disappear is always of great interest, but its practical value is greatly reduced if it does so only at a dose which eventually kills the animal, or has toxic side effects. The statement, once seen in a scientific publication, that animals died from the effects of the drug but were free from tumour, while interesting academically, would not inspire confidence in the use of the drug in man.

A tumour which was induced by a chemical in a rat in 1943, and has since been maintained by successive transplantations, can be used to demonstrate a procedure for testing for anti-cancer activity. Tiny fragments from the tumour of a donor animal are transplanted under the skin of a number of rats, taking care that the operation is carried out under sterile conditions. One week after the transplantation, all the rats will have readily noticeable tumours about 2 gm. in weight. At this time the animals are divided into seven groups. One group receives no treatment (the control group) but the other six groups are injected with the test drug. Different amounts of the drug are given to each rat of these test groups, and one week later the rats are killed and the tumours removed. Plate VI shows the tumours at this time, and how the ones from rats which received the drug compared with the control group which had not been treated. Groups 1 and 2 which had received only small amounts of the drug had tumours of a similar size to the control tumours, showing that the drug had no anti-cancer effect at these dose levels. There was a little effect in group 3, for the tumours were smaller than the controls, and in group 4 the tumours had not grown at all for they were the same size as they were a week earlier when the treatment had commenced. Group 5, given the second highest dose level of the drug, had no tumours. The drug at its highest dose, group 6, had killed all the rats before the end of the experiment. This test has answered the two questions required of it. In this system the new drug has anti-cancer activity and from the results, the difference in dose required to kill the tumour (dose 5) and to kill the animal (dose 6) can be calculated. This difference is often expressed as a ratio of the two doses and termed the therapeutic index.

In general anti-cancer agents have very poor therapeutic indices when compared with the indices of, for example, anti-bacterial agents.

The transplanted tumour taken for this example, named the Yoshida tumour after the Japanese doctor who first induced it, is used for only one of a great variety of similar tests for anti-cancer agents. The Cancer Chemotherapy National Service Center of America tests many hundreds of chemicals a year for their anti-cancer activity. At present, the first test for these chemicals is against a transplanted mouse leukaemia known as the L1210. This tumour has proved to be particularly valuable as a screening test. It is claimed that it would have detected every agent at present used clinically in the treatment of leukaemias and therefore is a reliable test for detecting new anti-leukaemic compounds. Unfortunately this does not mean that it will be just as reliable for predicting chemicals likely to be useful, for example, in the treatment of breast cancer.

Not only is this animal model a reliable test for anti-leukaemic agents but it has also been very valuable for studying in detail the behaviour of tumour cells on treatment with anti-cancer agents.

When mice are injected with the cells of this leukaemia they eventually die from the continued growth of the tumour. The time of death depends on the number of cells injected (see Table 1). If one thousand (10^3) tumour cells are given, the mice die twelve days later. A hundred times this number of cells (10^5), however, causes the animals to die at around eight days, and after 10 million cells (10^7) the animals die within six days. By measurement of the survival time of mice injected with a measured number of cells and then treated with a drug, a precise estimate can be made of the number of cancer cells that the drug

TABLE 1

Number of tumour cells injected	Average day of death
10,000,000 (10^7)	$5\frac{1}{2}$ days
1,000,000 (10^6)	7·0 days
100,000 (10^5)	8·0 days
10,000 (10^4)	10·0 days
1,000 (10^3)	12·0 days
100 (10^2)	13·0 days
1	14·0 days

The relationship between the number of L1210 tumour cells injected and the time it takes for the developing cancer to kill the mice.
[Adapted from : H. E. Skipper, F. M. Schabel and W. S. Wilcox, *Cancer Chem. Reports*, 1967]

163

has killed. Imagine that a group of mice have been injected with 1 million (10^6) leukaemic cells and then treated with a drug. Instead of dying at the expected time of seven days these animals may survive for ten days. Reference to Table 1 shows that ten days is the survival time for mice given 10,000 cells (10^4). In other words the chemical has reduced the effective number of

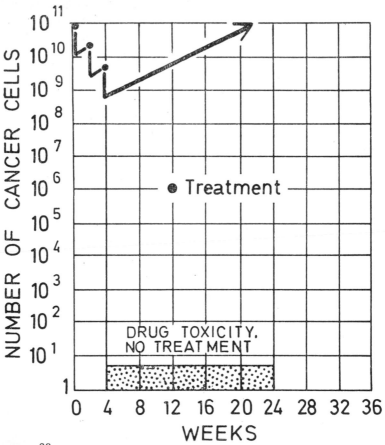

FIGURE 38

The patient is treated when his tumour consists of 10^{11} cells or about 100 gm. of tissue. Three treatments given over two weeks reduces the tumour to 1 gm. in size (10^9 cells). Treatment must be stopped at this point because of the drug's side effects. Before the next series of treatments can begin the tumour has regrown to a size greater than it was when first diagnosed. [Figures 38–41 and 46 are adapted from: J. K. Luce, G. P. Bodey and E. Frei, *Hospital Practice*, 1967.]

cancer cells injected from 1 million to 10,000. The drug has succeeded in killing 99 per cent of the tumour cell population.

This example incidentally illustrates how difficult it is to obtain a cure. Although the agent has succeeded in killing 99 per cent of the tumour cells in the mouse, the remaining cells continue to grow and eventually kill. Because there is no immune response against the few remaining cells the net result of therapy has not been a cure but slight extension of survival time.

From studies such as these we can now predict the ways in which sensitive human cancers will respond to chemotherapy. Figure 38 shows the most common type of response. A cancer has been detected when it consists of 10^{11} cells or about 100 gm. of tissue. In the example, treatment is given every two weeks until, at the end of the third treatment, the tumour is reduced in size to about 1 gm. (10^9 cells). This would be considered an extremely good response and at this time there would probably be no detectable symptoms of the presence of the tumour. However, as frequently happens, the drug must now be withheld because of its side effects. During the time that the drug is not given, the tumour regrows and when the patient is able to take more drug, the tumour may be larger than when it was first diagnosed. Even though the second course of chemotherapy may be just as effective as the first the tumour will never be eradicated because the amount by which it increases between treatments, is greater than the amount by which it is destroyed during the treatment. A cure is only possible if the cancer is so sensitive to the drug that several successive treatments can be given at non-toxic dose levels (Figure 39). The third or fourth administration of the drug will again lead to the apparent disappearance of the tumour, but treatment must be continued for another dozen courses or so to ensure that every cancer cell has been killed and the tumour does not regrow.

When a tumour responds so well to treatment, it is a problem to know when to stop treatment because the presence of less than 10 million (10^7) tumour cells will in most cases be quite undetectable. Only in the case of choriocarcinoma can such small quantities of tumour cells be detected. This tumour is highly sensitive to chemotherapy and responds in the manner of the example shown in Figure 39. The cells of this cancer excrete a chemical substance, gonadotrophin, which appears in

165

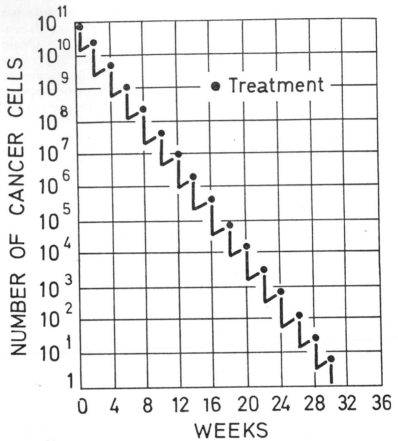

FIGURE 39

If a tumour is so sensitive to a chemical that several successive non-toxic doses of the drug are effective, it is necessary to continue treating for many weeks to ensure that every cancer cell is killed. The tumour would probably not be detectable once it has been reduced by treatment to about 10 million cells (10^7).

the urine and can be detected in very low concentrations. Treatment is continued until the level of this compound in the urine is reduced to normal levels. Sometimes as many as twelve intensive courses of treatment over many months needs to be given until the urinary gonadotrophin is normal and the patient is considered cured.

Figure 40 demonstrates the importance of detecting cancer

at an early stage. If many cancers could be detected when they only consisted of 10,000 cells or less, then probably sufficient courses of treatment could be given to kill every cancer cell before drug toxicity intervened.

Another type of response sometimes encountered is the development of resistance to treatment. Figure 41 shows that a tumour may initially respond well to treatment with an anti-cancer agent. However, this response decreases with successive

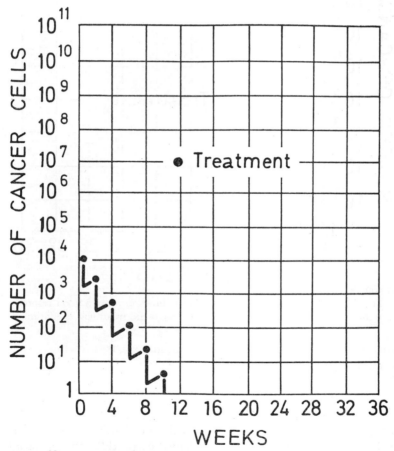

FIGURE 40

Early detection of a cancer means that a cure could be expected after a few courses of treatment. Sufficient doses of present day drugs could be given before toxicity intervenes.

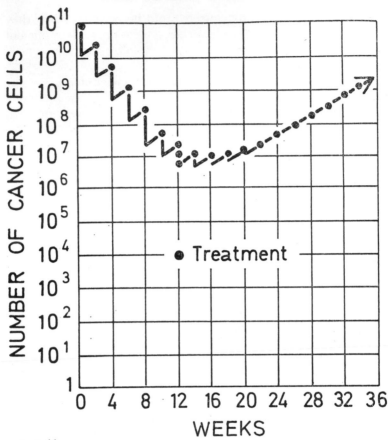

FIGURE 41

The development of resistance. A cancer shows initially a good response to treatment. Eventually it regrows even though the treatment is continued.

treatments until eventually the tumour starts growing again even though the drug is still being given.

OTHER SCREENING TESTS

In the screening of new antibiotics the need for animal models is bypassed by testing agents on cultures of different bacterial strains grown on dishes containing nutrients. In a similar way, cancer cells (human or animal) may be grown in culture and new chemicals screened against them for anti-cancer activity.

Past experience has shown, however, that this type of test is less reliable than those which use rats or mice with transplantable tumours. Where these and similar tests are used they serve as preliminary screens, the active compounds they detect being further tested on animals before being used in the clinic.

Figure 42 summarizes the different classes of chemical that were first shown to be effective on one or more animal tumours and then proved to be useful in the treatment of certain human cancers. The scheme shows that important cell chemicals, the nucleotides (see Chapter I), are formed from simple precursor molecules available in the cells. The different nucleotides are combined in an exact sequence to form a molecule of deoxyribo-nucleic acid (DNA). DNA controls the production of all the essential material that the cell needs both for its multiplication and for carrying out its normal functions. The enzymes which are responsible for the actual construction of the essential materials that the cell needs are themselves produced in structures known as the ribosomes. The production of each enzyme is controlled by a specific chemical, messenger RNA. When an enzyme is required for making a specific cell component,

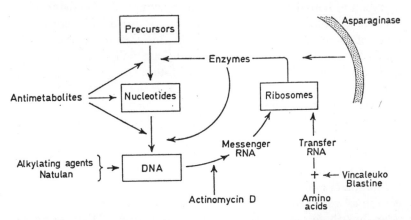

FIGURE 42
Scheme showing the ways in which the anti-cancer agents kill cells. Most of the chemicals are interfering with the synthesis of DNA.

169

messenger RNA is formed by the DNA molecule. The messenger RNA once it is formed moves to the ribosomes and initiates the synthesis of the appropriate enzyme. The amino acids of which the enzyme is composed are taken to the ribosomes by molecules of another chemical, transfer RNA. DNA can thus be seen to be controlling a sequence of events leading to the production of cell components as and when they are required. For a cancer to grow and eventually to kill there must, of course, be a continuous multiplication of cancer cells. Before a cell can divide it must duplicate all its DNA molecules so that each daughter cell will, after division, contain the exact amount of this regulatory chemical.

The Anti-Metabolites

The classes of agents, collectively called the anti-metabolites, interfere at some stage with the formation of nucleotides and so prevent the formation of the extra DNA required before cell division can take place. The anti-metabolites achieve this inhibition by being structurally similar to one of the precursor molecules (known as metabolites) which the enzymes build up to form the different nucleotides. The anti-metabolite, being so similar to the normal metabolite, is accepted by the enzyme. However, because of the slight change in structure the enzyme is prevented from converting it to the required compound and the anti-metabolite remains attached to the enzyme. The enzyme can, therefore, no longer carry out its function and if sufficient molecules of the enzyme are inactivated in this way the formation of the molecule that they normally produce will come to a halt and consequently DNA production will stop.

6-Mercaptopurine, used in the treatment of acute leukaemia, is a very powerful inhibitor of DNA synthesis. Figure 43 shows that this compound (abbreviated 6MP) is converted by the body to a nucleotide. The nucleotide so produced closely resembles a nucleotide found in the cell, inosinic acid, differing from it in only one atom. Inosinic acid is an essential intermediate in the formation of two nucleotide constituents of DNA. 6MP nucleotide combines very strongly with the enzymes that convert inosinic acid into these two nucleotides, and as a result DNA synthesis is prevented.

Knowing the chemical structure of the various intermediates

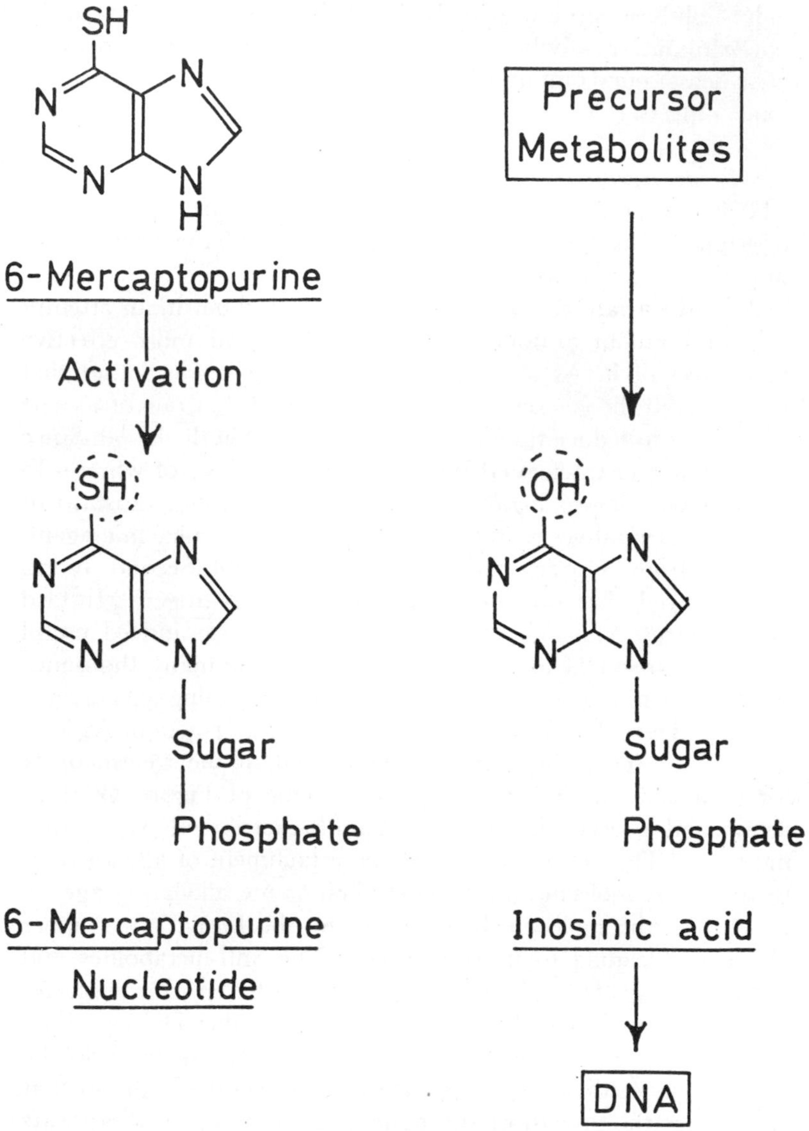

FIGURE 43

6-Mercaptopurine is converted to a nucleotide. This nucleotide is **very** similar to inosinic acid and prevents its conversion to nucleotides **required** for DNA production.

in DNA synthesis, the chemist makes related compounds differing only slightly in structure in the hope that they may prove to be powerful anti-metabolites. This approach has led to the discovery of at least four compounds highly effective in the treatment of some cancers.

Alkylating Agents

The first experience that the layman had of alkylating agents was during the First World War when one of these chemicals, sulphur mustard gas, was used with devastating effect as a biological warfare agent. Research was carried out in an attempt to find both an antidote to this war gas and more effective derivatives of it. As a result of this research it was found that not only did the gas burn severely on contact, but one of its side effects was to reduce the number of white cells in the blood. Since leukaemia is characterized by an excessive number of white cells in the blood, it was logically suggested that sulphur mustard or one of its derivatives might be useful as an anti-leukaemic agent. Reports from America published soon after the Second World War showed that one of these derivatives, Nitrogen Mustard (still referred to by its code name of HN2), was indeed useful in the treatment of leukaemia. Since that time many thousands of different nitrogen mustards and related alkylating agents have been synthesized and tested for their anti-cancer action. At least a dozen of these chemicals are now used in the treatment of some cancers. As indicated by the scheme of Figure 42 these agents and a recent discovery, Natulan, react directly with DNA molecules. This reaction involves the attachment of alkyl groups to the DNA molecule (and hence their name alkylating agents) preventing the molecule being used for the formation of more DNA and leading to its breakdown. The anti-metabolites and alkylating agents, although acting by different mechanisms, have the same end result – the inhibition of further DNA production and the prevention of cell multiplication. Not only do the cells no longer divide but they themselves eventually die so that not only is the growth of the cancer inhibited but it disappears completely.

It is perhaps difficult to imagine how chemicals as poisonous as the alkylating agents can ever kill cancer cells without harming normal cells. Some idea of how selective toxicity to cancer

172

cells can be achieved is demonstrated in Figure 44. In order to kill, an alkylating agent must penetrate the cell by crossing the cell wall. It must then travel through the cell to the nucleus where the DNA is situated. The chemical structure of the agent will determine whether it is readily transported across the cell walls or prevented from entering. The chemist endeavours to prepare structures which will readily be taken up by tumours but not by normal cells so that the poisonous substance is concentrated where it is required, i.e. in the cancer cell. In passing through

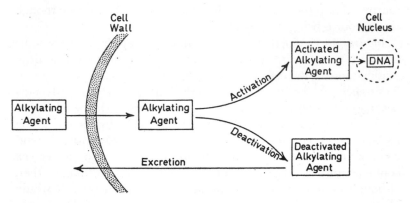

FIGURE 44

In order to kill cells an alkylating agent must cross the cell wall and reach DNA molecules in the cell nucleus. Its progress may be prevented by enzymes which either deactivate it, or fail to activate it, and by an impermeable cell wall.

the cell to the DNA in the nucleus the agent can be acted upon by enzymes so that it is converted to a structure that can no longer react with DNA. Such a deactivated form would then be excreted without damage to the cell. In this case the chemist tries to prepare agents which can be deactivated by enzymes which are present in normal cells but absent from cancer cells. Such an agent would obviously be selectively toxic to the cancer. Conversely the chemist can prepare so-called 'latent' alkylating agents. These are chemicals which are themselves non-toxic but which can be acted on by cellular enzymes to be converted into a toxic alkylating agent. Structures are designed which will be converted into toxic forms by cancer cells but not by normal cells.

173

In order to design such selective anti-cancer agents a lot must be known about the chemical make-up of cancer cells and how they differ from normal cells. The study of the chemistry of cancer cells is an important aspect of present day cancer research.

In practice such perfect selectivity of action is never achieved. Even the best anti-metabolites and alkylating agents have serious side effects caused by destruction of normal tissues. Bone marrow cells are continually dividing to replace the red and white cells of the blood which only have a short existence. This dividing tissue is also susceptible to these agents, and it is damage to bone marrow that often makes the clinician stop treatment even though the tumour is being destroyed.

Figure 44 incidentally shows how a cancer may become resistant to a drug. A cancer may initially transport a drug readily across its cell wall and so be very susceptible to it. Resistance to the drug will develop if the cancer cells now became relatively impermeable to the agent. If the chemical used was a 'latent' agent, resistance would arise by the cell losing its activating enzymes and no longer converting the 'latent' compound to its active form. On the other hand, a cancer cell could acquire a large amount of deactivating enzyme so that, although large quantities of the agent entered the cell, it would all be deactivated and excreted before reacting with DNA.

Other Anti-cancer Agents
Actinomycin D and Vincaleukoblastine are two naturally occurring chemicals, the former isolated from a mould and the latter from the periwinkle plant. Both these compounds inhibit DNA synthesis in an indirect way. Actinomycin D is a very complicated structure but of such a precise shape that it interlocks exactly with a DNA molecule. This prevents the formation of the messenger RNAs and, therefore, the synthesis of enzymes required for further DNA synthesis is inhibited. Vincaleukoblastine has the same end result but it achieves this by preventing amino acids being attached to transfer RNA and taken to the ribosomes where they are assembled to form enzymes.

The discovery of the anti-tumour effect of asparaginase, itself an enzyme, is one of the most exciting recent discoveries in cancer chemotherapy. It is now known that certain cancers require the amino acid asparagine, presumably for the assembly of certain enzymes and other cell components. This amino acid is, therefore, essential to this type of cancer. However, for normal cells the amino acid is not essential because they can produce it from simple precursors available in the cell. Cancers requiring this compound survive and grow because, like true parasites, they take it up from the bloodstream where it has been excreted by normal cells. The enzyme asparaginase converts the amino acid into another derivative of no use to the cancer. By administering the enzyme so that it circulates in the blood all the asparagine is removed. As a result the cancer can no longer obtain its supply of this essential foodstuff and it rapidly dies. The beauty of this form of chemotherapy is that the agent is not toxic to the host because no normal cell requires the amino acid. Asparaginase has now been prepared in pure form and clinical trials at present in progress indicate that in combination with other agents it is effective in the treatment of acute leukaemia. Unfortunately many other cancers are not sensitive to this drug because presumably they can make their own asparagine.

The discovery of the anti-tumour effect of this enzyme arose by pure chance when guinea pig serum, which is very rich in asparaginase, was administered to mice with tumours which required asparagine as an essential amino acid. Other tumours may exist deficient in one nutrient or another which they obtain from the host. By extensive studies of the chemistry of different cancer cells or by pure chance as described above for asparaginase, we will eventually come to know more about the ways in which cancers may differ from normal tissues. A knowledge of these differences will then enable us to design drugs which are selectively toxic to cancers.

DRUG ADMINISTRATION

Certain principles for the administration of drugs have always been recognized. Actinomycin D, for example, which is very sensitive to acid, is always given by injection into a vein and not by mouth because by the latter route it would be destroyed by the acid of the stomach before reaching the cancer. Only recently, however, it has been realized that, for much more subtle reasons, both the route by which some drugs are given and the dosage schedule chosen (i.e. daily or weekly for example) can profoundly

175

affect their anti-cancer activity. These facts were first detected by using animal models, and then shown to also apply to man.

Table 2 compares the anti-leukaemic effect of the anti-metabolite cytosine arabinoside in mice when given by two different dosage schedules. The first dosage schedule employed the drug every four days at a dose of 240 mg/kg. No mice were cured and at the end of treatment there were 10^9 (one thousand million) leukaemic cells left, indicating that the drug was not very effective. In the second dosage schedule the drug was given in smaller quantities but more frequently, eight times a day on every fourth day. At the end of the treatment every tumour cell was killed and the mice were cured. In both cases as much of the drug as possible had been given (the amount of drug causing toxicity is dependent on the dosage schedule) but whereas the first dosage schedule was of little value the second dosage schedule gave complete cures.

TABLE 2

Dose mg/kg	Time of Injections	Total Dose	Number of Animals Cured	Leukaemic Cells at end of Treatment
240	2, 6, 10, 14 days	960	0/10	10^9
15	8 times daily on days 2, 6, 10, 14	480	10/10	None

The effect of the antimetabolite cytosine arabinoside on the growth of the L1210 leukaemia. The first dose schedule has little effect but the second dose schedule is curative.
[Adapted from : H. E. Skipper, F. M. Schabel and W. S. Wilcox, *Cancer Chem. Reports*, 1967]

Similar experiments on tumour bearing animals have shown that the anti-tumour effect of some drugs can be dramatically changed by altering the route of administration. If the nitrogen mustard HN2 is given to rats with a Walker tumour by injection

176

into a vein in the leg, it kills the animal at a dose of about 1·5 mg/kg. but causes complete regression of the tumour at 1/15th of this dose (0·1 mg/kg.) (Table 3). However if the compound is injected into the vein leading to the liver it is no longer effective in killing the tumour but is just as toxic to the animal.

TABLE 3

INTRAVENOUS		INTRA-PORTAL	
Tumour curative dose	Toxic dose	Tumour curative dose	Toxic dose
0·1 mg/kg.	1·5 mg/kg.	None	1·8 mg/kg.

HN2 when given intravenously can cause regression of a rat tumour at 1/15th of the toxic dose. If given by the intra-portal vein so that it passes through the liver before reaching the tumour, it is just as toxic but has no effect on the tumour.
[Adapted from : L. M. Cobb, *Int. J. Cancer*, 1966]

Figure 45 demonstrates how these findings in the laboratory are applied with benefit to man. If children with acute leukaemia are given the anti-metabolite methotrexate, daily by mouth, less than one-fifth of them remain free from symptoms for longer than twenty-four weeks. However, if the same drug is given by a different route (into the muscle instead of by mouth) and by a different dosage schedule (larger amounts weekly instead of daily) the response is very much better. More than half of the children so treated remain free of symptoms of the disease for longer than forty-eight weeks. For each drug there probably exists an optimum route of administration and dosage schedule. Further work on animal models will almost certainly improve the results obtained in the clinic with the anti-cancer agents we already have available.

Drugs in Combination
Quite often, when a patient is responding well to treatment, administration of the agent has to be discontinued because of

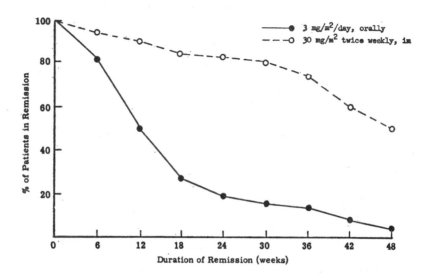

Comparative Effects of Two Dose Schedules of Methotrexate on Remission Duration in Acute Leukemia in Children.

FIGURE 45
A comparison of the effectiveness of the anti-metabolite methotrexate given in two different ways in the treatment of acute leukaemia. The conventional method uses methotrexate daily given by mouth. In terms of length of survival free from symptoms of leukaemia, this schedule is much less effective than methotrexate given by injection into the muscle and twice weekly. [*Cancer Chem. Reports,* **50** (1966).]

side effects, so allowing the cancer to recover and regrow. A second agent could be administered at this time if the side effects it produced were of a different nature to the side effects of the first drug and therefore not cumulative. The sequential administration of two or more drugs, termed combination chemotherapy, has achieved results far better than the administration of either drug alone in the treatment of some cancers. Prednisone, a steroid, and asparaginase for instance do not produce as a major side effect the damage to bone marrow that is seen with the alkylating agents, anti-metabolites, vincaleukoblastine and actinomycin D and can profitably be used in combination with these agents.

In the treatment of acute leukaemia in children a drug is first administered in attempts to remove the symptoms of the disease (excessive number of white cells in the blood and abnormal cells in the bone marrow) and return the patient to good health. This first stage of treatment is termed induction. Past experience has shown that even after the disappearance of all signs of the tumour the patient will often relapse once more with the symptoms of leukaemia. The time of this relapse can be delayed considerably and sometimes the patient cured, by treatment (or maintenance) during the time when no signs of the leukaemia are present. Several compounds are known which are effective in induction causing disappearance of symptoms of the disease and other agents are known which are effective in maintaining this remission once it has been induced.

Using a single drug, between 21 and 57 per cent of patients with acute leukaemia undergo remission. However, if drug combinations such as the anti-metabolites cytosine arabinoside

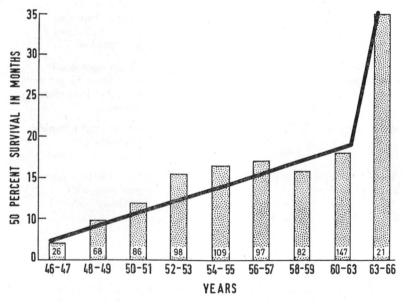

FIGURE 46

Progress in the treatment of acute leukaemia by chemotherapy. Since 1944 considerable progress has been made by the discovery of new agents and by their more effective use in combination and at optimum dose schedules.

179

or 6-mercaptopurine are given in conjunction with either prednisone or asparaginase up to 90 per cent of patients undergo remission. The length of remission can then be considerably increased by employing further drug combinations during the period of remission.

Our progress in the treatment of this cancer is well illustrated in Figure 46. In the 1940s, after acute leukaemia had been diagnosed, the average survival time was about two months. At the present day, because of the more effective agents, their use under optimum conditions and in combination, the mean survival

TABLE 4

Cancers which respond best to Chemotherapy

DISEASE	TREATMENT	RESPONSE
Choriocarcinoma	Methotrexate Actinomycin D Vincaleukoblastine	80 per cent complete remission of disease. Probable cures in all cases of remission
Burkitt's Lymphoma	Alkylating agents	60 per cent good remissions. 15 per cent complete long-term remissions
Wilms tumour	X-rays and Actinomycin D in combination	80 per cent complete remission with long-term survival
Acute Leukaemia in Children	Combinations of Prednisone and Asparaginase with Alkylating agents, Anti-metabolites, and Vincaleuko-blastine	90 per cent complete remission with increased survival time

If treatment causes the cancer to disappear with no remaining symptoms of its presence, the patient is in complete remission. This complete remission must be maintained for many years before the patient can be considered cured. Remissions are classified as partial, good, complete, etc.

time from diagnosis is now thirty-two months with the possibility of complete cure. With such progress it is not too much to hope that in the near future deaths from this cancer may be prevented completely.

Today at least three cancer types may be treated by chemotherapy with high hopes of a cure (Table 4).

CHAPTER IX

HORMONES AND CANCER

R. D. BULBROOK

HORMONES IN GENERAL

Hormones are chemical 'messengers' that are synthesized in specialized tissues such as the ovaries, testes, adrenal glands, pituitary gland and pancreas. In response to certain stimuli such as low blood-sugar level, heat and cold, etc., they are released into the blood stream and carried to their 'target' organs. The hormones control absolutely the growth and function of some target tissues but in others they may exert only minor effects.

There are about forty different hormones, each with an important and specific function. Some are complicated protein molecules consisting of long chains of amino acids arranged in a definite pattern. Insulin, the hormone that controls the level of sugar in the blood, is of this type. The 'steroids' make up another large group of hormones. These are relatively simple compounds with either 18, 19 or 21 carbon atoms arranged in four rings which form the steroid nucleus. The biological activities of the steroids depend upon the nature of additional groups of atoms attached to the nucleus. Very slight differences in these substituent groups result in enormous changes in physiological activity. For example, oestradiol is the main female sex hormone yet it differs from testosterone (the male sex hormone) only in having 1 carbon atom and 4 hydrogen atoms fewer.

A striking feature shared by most hormones is their great biological activity in very low concentrations: the blood level of oestradiol in a normal young woman is about 0·000,000,06 of a gramme in 100 millilitres of blood, yet this is enough to maintain normal breast, uterine and vaginal, structure and function.

There are some twenty active compounds in the steroid group

that are produced naturally in the endocrine organs (the ductless glands) and several thousand different steroid-like compounds that have been synthesized by the organic chemists.

The steroids are classified mainly on the basis of their biological functions. The groups are: the corticosteroids, made in the adrenal cortex and controlling sugar metabolism and salt and water balance; the female sex hormones (the oestrogens and progestins) made in the ovaries and placenta and controlling growth and function of the breast and uterus; and the male sex hormones (the androgens), controlling such things as prostate and seminal vesicle growth and function, hair growth and, to a limited extent, muscle mass.

The reason for dealing with the steroid hormones at such length is that most of the research work on the relation between hormones and cancer has been carried out with these compounds.

HORMONES AND NORMAL BREAST GROWTH

It might be helpful to examine the actions of a variety of hormones on one particular tissue (the breast) as an example of how hormones work. In the new-born mammal, the breast consists of a few minor passageways (ducts) lined with epithelial cells. Without hormonal stimuli, the breast would remain in this rudimentary state. As the animal matures, a variety of hormones act in sequence. In most animals, the oestrogens and progesterone act together to cause a rapid and dramatic proliferation of the ducts, in much the same way as a seedling pushes its root system through the surrounding soil. If the animal becomes pregnant, two pituitary hormones take over; growth hormone and prolactin. Buds form on the side of the ducts and then the buds hollow out to form sacs. The cells lining these sacs have the task of manufacturing and secreting milk. Groups of sacs are formed into bundles with a large main duct. The detailed processes are comparable to those in a ship-building yard, with thousands of components being required at the right place at the right time. The hormones might be compared with an (efficient) board of directors.

During the changes from a rudimentary duct system to a lactating mammary gland the number of cells increases by many

183

million-fold. Hormones other than those mentioned above play subsidiary roles.

It has to be admitted that we do not know a great deal about the way hormones bring about these changes (and, of all the mammals, we know least about women). It now seems that the target tissues possess special binding sites which capture the hormones as they pass in the circulating blood. When the hormones are bound, biological action ensues. How this happens is one of the great problems of endocrinology.

OTHER HORMONE-DEPENDENT OR SENSITIVE TISSUES

Breast growth is one of the most dramatic examples of hormone action but growth and function of many other organs are either absolutely or partially dependent on hormonal stimuli. Among them are the uterus, vagina, prostate, and seminal vesicles. Little more will be said about cancers in these organs since the main body of research work has to do with breast cancer.

HORMONES AND CANCER

If hormones can have such a profound influence on cell growth, can they push the cells one stage further into uncontrolled and continuous growth which is basically the property of most tumours? There is still no evidence that the hormones cause the actual transformation from a normal to a malignant cell but in one sense they might be considered as carcinogens. Suppose malignant change is a random event affecting cells with a frequency of one in a million. If hormones increase the number of cells at risk by a factor of ten, then ten times as many cancers will occur. In one sense, the hormones are not the 'causative agents' (which could be viruses) but in practical terms their importance is obvious.

What we do know with absolute certainty is that, if certain hormones are administered to laboratory animals in large doses over long periods of time, many cancers appear that are not present in untreated controls. The list of such experimental cancers is a long one and covers many species of animals. Cancers have been induced in the breast, uterus, kidneys, blood cells (leukaemia), adrenal glands, ovaries, thyroid and pituitary gland by such means.

HORMONES AND CANCER IN MAN

The first real evidence that some human cancers could be influenced by hormones was obtained before hormones were discovered! In the middle of the nineteenth century, a young Scottish doctor, George Beatson, found himself a splendid job looking after a feeble-minded boy on a remote estate. His duties were light and he became interested in the processes leading to lactation in sheep. In particular, he was impressed by the remarkable similarities between the appearance of the rapidly growing mammary gland and that of breast cancer in women. He also knew that breast function in sheep was dependent on normal ovarian activity.

Many years later, Beatson saw two women in Glasgow with hopelessly advanced breast cancer. He reasoned that removal of their ovaries might remove an essential stimulus to the breast tissue and possibly to the tumour arising from it. He decided to see what would happen if the patients' ovaries were removed and, in the event, found a dramatic improvement in one of his patients, with the virtual disappearance of the tumour. This work was published in the *Lancet* in 1896. Removal of the ovaries in young women remains a standard treatment of advanced breast cancer to this day.

The attack on well-established tumours by the removal of glands that secrete substances which stimulate or support tumour growth has been much developed in the last twenty-five years. Charles Huggins, in Chicago, showed that any method that would bring about atrophy of the normal prostate gland in animals was also effective in controlling prostatic cancer in some of his patients. This finding destroyed the idea that all cancers were independent growths and emphasized that at least some tumours were still dependent on normal control mechanisms. Huggins then extended Beatson's early findings on the beneficial effects of oophorectomy on breast cancer. He and his colleagues had evidence that the adrenal glands also produced hormones that stimulated breast and prostatic tumour growth and they went on to show that removal of the adrenals could lead to

185

great clinical benefit in some patients. Subsequently, Swedish workers obtained similar results following removal of the pituitary gland (hypophysectomy). The adrenal glands will not function in the absence of the pituitary gland and hypophysectomy also leads to the removal of pituitary hormones that have a direct action on breast tissues.

Hormonal treatments are almost invariably used for patients with, what is loosely termed, 'advanced' disease. In 'early' breast cancer, the tumour is localized in the breast. If treatment is carried out in time, the tumour and the surrounding normal tissue are removed surgically and a complete cure is effected. But in some patients, the tumour has already started to spread by the time the first diagnosis is made. This means that groups of cells have broken away from the original tumour and travelled in the blood or lymph stream to distant parts of the body where they lodge and multiply. At first, these new centres of growth are undetectable but as time goes on they may become as big as the original tumour. If there are a few well-defined secondary growths, they may be destroyed by X-ray therapy or by surgical removal but sometimes there are multiple sites of growth. Patients with such secondary growths are said to have the 'advanced' disease.

It is an unfortunate fact that removal of endocrine organs only brings about marked clinical benefit in about a third of the patients with advanced breast cancer. Perhaps another third get some slight benefit, mainly in relief of pain. In the remainder, the disease is unchecked. Even in those who do well, relief may only be transient.

There are two theories to account for the temporary nature of the effects of treatment by removal of sources of hormones. The first is that not all cancer cells are killed and the survivors become altered in such a way that they can continue to grow in a hostile hormone environment. The other is that the tumour already consists of a mixture of different populations of cells by the time treatment is carried out – some populations are hormone dependent, others are not. After treatment, the dependent cells die and the independent cells take over.

A final paradox must be mentioned. In the last thirty years it has been found that administration of huge amounts of steroid hormones may also lead to tumour regression. Stilboestrol (a

186

synthetic oestrogen) and testosterone were the first to be used. In the last ten years there has been an intensive search for better compounds, so far without success, although some of the newer drugs have fewer side-effects.

THE SELECTION OF PATIENTS FOR THERAPY

In most hospitals, the treatment of patients with advanced breast cancer follows a set pattern. If the patient is pre-menopausal, the ovaries are removed. If, and when, this treatment fails, hormones are administered by mouth or by injection. If the tumour continues to grow, adrenalectomy is carried out. In a few centres hypophysectomy may be done but this operation requires good neurosurgical facilities. Almost all patients are treated in this way because there has been no method of selecting responsive cases and sparing unresponsive ones from unnecessary major surgery. In the last few years a test has been discovered which makes the selection of suitable cases a practical proposition. Workers in England, France, Japan and America have shown that responsive patients excrete in their urine normal amounts of products derived from the male sex hormones (the androgen metabolites) where unresponsive patients excrete subnormal amounts. The reason for this association between the androgens and the clinical course of breast cancer is completely obscure but the practical advantages of such a test are obvious.

What is of more importance is that the finding of such an association between natural hormone production and the way a tumour responded to treatment prompted a wider search for similar correlations in patients with less widespread disease and eventually in the normal population itself.

EARLY BREAST CANCER

In the majority of cases, cancer is first noticed as a lump in the breast. (Most lumps in the breast are benign and the diagnosis of cancer can only be made after the lump has been removed and studied under a microscope.) By the time diagnosis is made, some patients will show evidence that cells from the tumour have started migration to distant parts of the body (the new tumour colonies are called metastases). Generally speaking, the lymph nodes in the arm-pit are the first to be involved. The operation of radical mastectomy is used to remove the breast, the tumour within, and the lymph nodes.

There is a great deal of argument about the true cure rate from this treatment, but the majority of patients survive five to ten years without further symptoms. Nevertheless, there remains the acute clinical problem that some patients have a very rapid recurrence of their disease after mastectomy and there is no way of identifying the group before operation.

Recently, some evidence has been obtained that this high-risk group are characterized by precisely the same abnormality that was found in some patients with the advanced disease : that is, patients with a high rate of recurrence after mastectomy tend to excrete subnormal amounts of androgen metabolites in their urine. This has led to an international trial of methods of additional treatment at mastectomy that might slow down renewed tumour growth. Some form of selection is needed in such preventative treatment since to give all patients additional treatment would mean that many of them who were completely cured of their disease by mastectomy would be given treatments that carried some risk or had unpleasant side-effects.

THE PRE-CLINICAL PERIOD IN BREAST CANCER

The finding that some patients with early breast cancer have a pronounced abnormality in their urinary steroid excretion raises an interesting point. Does the presence of a small tumour, often no bigger than a pea, lead to alterations in the secretion of the relevant hormones or do the hormonal abnormalities have anything to do with the genesis of the tumour? It ought to be emphasized at this point that, by the time a breast tumour is diagnosed, some two-thirds of its life span has already been passed. If a tumour starts as a single cell, the first cell division would give 2 cells : each of these would divide to give 4 cells. These would give 8 cells; then 16, 32, 64, 128 and so on. Each wave of division may be followed by a month of quiescence so that a considerable period of time would be required for an aggregation of 100 million cells to form, and this is a number that would give a visible or palpable lump. Although the time scale may be long, only thirty waves of divisions of the original cell and its progeny would be required. Once a visible tumour is found only a few more divisions would be required (about ten or fifteen) to form a huge tumour mass weighing several pounds, if the disease were to be left untreated.

It has been calculated that the time from one cell to 100 million cells may average about ten years in breast cancer. If the change from a normal to a malignant cell is caused by an abnormal hormone environment or if the speed at which cell divisions occur is controlled by hormonal factors, then we have to look for these changes in women in their early thirties because it is about ten years later that incidence starts to rise sharply.

PROSPECTIVE STUDIES

The only way to check whether abnormal hormone production precedes the clinical appearance of breast cancer is to carry out a prospective study. This means examining various aspects of the hormonal environment in a large and ostensibly normal population and then waiting until a proportion of the volunteers appear with the disease. Their previous hormone records can then be checked to see whether abnormalities existed before the disease was diagnosed.

An investigation of this nature has been in progress in the Imperial Cancer Research Fund and at Guy's Hospital for the last eight years. Although breast cancer is the commonest cancer in women and eventually affects 1 in 25, its incidence is spread over a long time. The rate in women aged 35–55 years is about one in 800 per year. Therefore, a normal population of some 5,000 volunteers might be expected to yield about six cases of breast cancer each year.

The investigation in question is being carried out in Guernsey. In this small island there is a tight-knit, stable population of some 45,000 people with a strong community spirit. This has made possible the collection of complete 24-hour urine specimens from 5,000 volunteers. Almost equally important, there are few doctors and one hospital, so that no cases of cancer among the volunteers go unreported. The urines have been frozen to $-20°C$. and flown to London for processing. Since the actual chemical measurement of the androgen breakdown products is a difficult analytical procedure, a crude urine extract has been made and

189

stored. When a case of breast cancer is reported amongst the volunteers, the analysis of her androgen metabolites is taken to completion together with those of ten matched controls (normal women without the disease). If the thesis that women with breast cancer have abnormal steroid levels before diagnosis is correct, then the analytical results on the cancer case should differ from those found for the controls.

A preliminary report indicates that about two-thirds of the cases of breast cancer so far reported from Guernsey had hormonal abnormalities before their diseases became manifest.

EARLY DIAGNOSIS

If the first results of the Guernsey experiment can be substantiated, it is possible that hormone assays might provide a means of identifying a group of apparently normal women who have a high risk of breast cancer. There is already a new technique for detecting very small breast tumours. This is a special type of X-ray examination known as mammography, and by this means tumours can be found that could not possibly have been detected by normal clinical methods.

The hope is that early operation in patients found by this technique will mean that the tumours are removed before they have had time to disseminate to other parts of the body. Whether this will really be an effective weapon in terms of increasing the cure rate from mastectomy remains to be seen. However, it might be extremely useful in combination with hormone assays.

Ideally, it would be preferable to go back even further in the life span of the tumour, to the point where it would be completely undetectable by any conceivable physical means, and to attempt to correct the basic endocrine abnormalities. But the sad fact is that we are still uncertain about the hormonal changes that lead to the abnormalities in the excretion of androgen breakdown products. The hormonal environment can be compared with a railway marshalling yard. If one wagon is shunted into another, the effects reverberate down the rest of the train. If there is a buffer, the shock wave passes all the way back again. Similarly, it is almost impossible to alter the level of one hormone without affecting either the level or the physiological actions of several others.

The original Guernsey findings are being followed up by a second prospective study in which the blood steroids (especially the precursors of the urinary androgen metabolites) are being measured. In Holland, a prospective study is examining the oestrogen levels. These investigations may throw more light on the underlying endocrine lesions.

FUTURE POSSIBILITIES

There is always the hope that a fortuitous discovery could transform the treatment of breast cancer and other hormone-related cancers overnight. After all, people do win fortunes on Football Pools, at astronomical odds. However, most of us do not plan our lives on the supposition that such a windfall will come our way and it is much more likely that advances in the prevention and treatment of hormone dependent cancers will stem from research now being pursued all over the world or from new lines developing from present results.

In terms of surgical treatment of either early or advanced breast and prostatic cancer, little advance can be expected. Hormonal treatment by removal of endocrine organs might improve marginally if selection procedures are designed to tailor the available treatments to the patient's individual needs. With the synthesis of so many new compounds, administration of large doses of steroids or steroid-like compounds has some hope of future advance but, after intensive work over the last twenty years, no compound has emerged that is clearly superior to the steroids first used thirty years ago.

The main hope at the moment must lie in earlier diagnosis, coupled with earlier treatment. Ultimately, the identification and correction of basic endocrine abnormalities, or manipulation of the endocrine environment holds the greatest promise. That day is still a long way off.

CHAPTER X

THE CONTROL OF CANCER IN THE FUTURE

J. Q. MATTHIAS

The last century has seen in great measure the conquest of disease due to infection by bacteria. Effective forms of treatment, particularly the antibiotics, have been discovered, and successful preventive measures such as isolation and immunization have been developed. Smaller numbers dying from infectious diseases necessarily means an increase in number of those exposed to the risk of developing a cancer. Nowadays, in some communities, as many as 1 in 3 or 4 develop cancer in some form and 1 in 5 may die as a consequence. In most instances the increase is the inevitable result of the dramatic increase in life expectancy evident in recent years. Only in a few specialized sites, notably the lung, the bladder and the blood, is the actual risk increasing demonstrably.

The effective control of cancer is in greater part a hope of the future; nevertheless *much can* be accomplished *today*. Any consideration of possible ways of controlling the disease must include what is known of prevention, in the passive sense of avoiding known or suspected causes; the possibilities of active prevention or prophylaxis; as well as means of achieving early diagnosis and effective treatment both of the pre-cancerous state and the developed malignancy.

It is not always necessary to know the precise details of the aetiology of a disease before effective means of control are possible. Jenner, when he used cow-pox vaccination to protect men against smallpox, did not know that the two diseases were caused by viruses sufficiently similar to allow one to protect against the other. He realized that persons who had had cow-pox never developed the more serious disease; an observation which led him to take the major forward step of deliberately infecting a normal fit human being with the contents of cow-pox pustules to prevent the subsequent development of smallpox. Cancer is, unfortunately, a far more baffling and complex problem. It is not a single disease but many different diseases caused by many factors, only some of which are known. Nevertheless, more is known about the causes of some types of cancers than about many non-cancerous conditions! Some cancers can be prevented, many can be cured; in other cases the difficulty is not a lack of knowledge but in its application!

The enormous amount of scientific data about the cancer problem and the characteristics of tumour cells is confusing, and frequently appears contradictory. It is likely that a basically similar change is responsible for the behaviour of all tumour cells but that this change may be brought about in a number of different ways. There is in all probability a final common pathway linking genetic, viral, chemical and physical carcinogenesis. At the practical level of cause and effect, steps towards cancer prevention can, and must, begin without a detailed knowledge of fundamental mechanisms.

The primary change responsible for the malignancy results in other disorders of the cancer cells which may confuse by appearing to be intimately concerned with the malignant change, although only, in fact, by-products. Some of the parallel, or accessory, features may however contribute to the recognition of the cell as abnormal by the body and therefore, in some circumstances, to its elimination. Some point out that the aberration of growth control which we know as cancer cannot be fully appreciated until the precise details of normal growth are understood. To some extent this is so. However our ignorance of normal growth control mechanisms must not be made an excuse for failing to study the cancer cell *in situ*, which will, without doubt, throw important light on the control of normal growth.

Mechanisms developed during evolution to protect the body against invasion by foreign (antigenic) material, including bacteria and cells, may have had their origins in mechanisms designed to eliminate aberrations in its own cells. Cancer cells may have lost tissue-specific substances or antigens and may no longer be subject to tissue homeostatic control mechanisms. The body either no longer recognizes the tendency to overgrowth as

N 193

a threat or is unable to respond sufficiently. The loss of tissue-specific antigen may be brought about by any of countless means. There is good evidence that cells of lymphoid origin are able to recognize antigenic, or structural, changes and are able actively to discourage, and indeed to eliminate, them. Experimentally stimulation of the system responsible for immunity in the body delays the appearance of induced and grafted tumours and depression of that system facilitates their growth. Perhaps displaced, or aged, tissue is removed by a mechanism which shares features with that influencing tumours possessing distinct abnormal antigens.

An interesting property of cancer cells is their lack of sensitivity to the inhibiting presence of neighbouring cells. The cellular contacts between tumour cells are often faulty; a phenomenon known as a failure of contact inhibition, and thought to be the result of changes in the cell surface.

A chalone is a substance produced locally which inhibits cell division. It is possible that the concentration of these substances may fall in cancerous states and so permit continued growth. If these substances could be isolated they might have a potential for treatment particularly as they would be physiological and probably relatively non-toxic. The greater danger of malignant changes in ectopic tissue than in the same tissue in its rightful place indicates that the absence of tissue control factors is possibly of the highest importance.

Elucidation of the ways in which multicellular organisms recognise and eliminate abnormal cells and control growth is one of the most pressing needs of cancer research today. Initially many tumours appear to be of limited malignancy. Later they become more malignant (more resistant to normal mechanisms of control). Some tumours are at the outset sensitive to natural hormones, but later completely resistant. If the biological mechanisms accounting for such striking changes could be understood, we would be a long way towards developing means of influencing the inevitable progress towards autonomous, relentless growth.

The steps which might be taken to protect man from the known carcinogenic hazards of his environment have been outlined in a previous chapter. This chapter will be concerned with the advances which might be expected in therapy.

TREATMENT

The current, proven methods of treating malignant disease are by surgery, radiotherapy and chemotherapy. Surgery and radiotherapy are both capable of cure in favourable circumstances, and both able to relieve symptoms when cure is no longer possible. Cure is a word which must be used circumspectly in relation to cancer. There is no way of being absolutely sure that all malignant cells are eliminated by any form of treatment and, as it is well known, in certain malignancies undoubted secondaries or metastases may declare themselves fifteen or twenty years after an apparent cure. The approach to cure can only be understood in terms of the percentage of patients free of clinical disease after treatment. For convenience the survival rates are usually quoted at intervals of five years; so one speaks of five-year, ten-year, and fifteen-year cures. The accepted sure way of 'curing' cancer is to remove it in its entirety.

Surgery

Modern advances in surgical and anaesthetic technique, resuscitation and patient care, have made major surgery relatively safe so that the limitations imposed nowadays are physiological rather than anatomical. Future developments lie particularly in the replacement of the organs involved. Already lung and liver transplants are being attempted and possibly other organs (e.g. pancreas) will be attempted later.

Radiotherapy

Radiotherapy on the other hand depends, for its cures, on its ability to destroy cancer cells *in situ*. Major advances in techniques have made possible the administration of radiation doses sufficient to kill tumour cells in some circumstances, without unacceptable damage to the skin, bone and adjacent tissue. Cures are regularly achieved in cancer of the skin, testes and Hodgkin's disease but, unfortunately, less commonly in other tumours.

The fact that there is no way of detecting a small number of cancer cells means that the disease could well have escaped beyond its original confines and therefore be incurable in terms of surgery or radiotherapy. It is in this sort of case, overtly amenable to cure, that chemotherapy is being used in clinical trials in combination with surgery and/or radiotherapy. It is hoped that a course of systemic treatment will either eliminate, or substantially reduce, the numbers of any malignant cells which may have escaped beyond the local site of origin. Possibly their numbers may be reduced sufficiently to allow the natural, immunological responses of the body to complete their elimination. Examples of tumours in which it seems worthwhile combining chemotherapy with surgery or radiotherapy are Wilms' tumour and neuroblastoma in children. Possibly also in Hodgkin's disease the outlook is improved by the addition of chemotherapy to radiotherapy; and in carcinoma of the breast by a combination of surgery and chemotherapy.

Chemotherapy

The treatment of cancer by drugs alone cannot, at the present time, be said, except for a few rare tumours, to cure. In the overwhelming majority of cancers, the role of chemotherapy is still confined to inoperable, incurable, disseminated cancers. Unfortunately current drugs are rarely able to eradicate every cancer cell in the body. Their side effects are so marked as to limit severely the amounts that can be given.

It is, however, in the sphere of the treatment of cancer medically that the most exciting advances are being made. Until recently, no drug was known which would destroy cancer cells specifically. Inevitably normal tissues were also affected. The most susceptible tissues are those in which the cells divide most frequently such as the bone marrow (red and white cell precursors), intestinal tract, the germ cells and the hair follicles. Advances in the treatment of cancer by drugs are proceding along two channels: first, the development of new drugs with anti-cancer properties; and secondly, the better use of those presently available. Possibly the most exciting and significant discovery of recent years has been the demonstration of the effect of the enzyme asparaginase on certain cancer cells. Tumours susceptible to the enzyme have been found to lack the ability to synthesize an amino acid called asparagine (see p. 174). It is believed that the enzyme depletes the body of asparagine and thus denies the malignant cell an essential metabolite. This epoch-making discovery is the first convincing demonstration of a qualitative biochemical difference between normal and cancer cells. Normal cells are able to synthesize asparagine from simple precursors but certain cancer cells cannot. Thus the administration of the enzyme prevents cancer cells from growing but does not interfere with the division of normal cells.

The development and manufacture of asparaginase is in much the same stage today as was that of penicillin in the early 1940s. It is very expensive, in very short supply, and as might be expected, it is also impure. Thus, the amounts that are given are not only limited by the availability of the drug, but also by its side effects. The enzyme, derived commercially from bacteria, acts as a foreign protein and its administration may be followed by sensitization. In the doses which are being given at present, its benefits are strictly limited. The only tumours sensitive with any uniformity are certain leukaemias in children. Unfortunately it is already clear that it is unlikely that any tumour in man can be completely eradicated by the enzyme. Its importance, however, lies in its mode of action and in the stimulus given to the search for other exploitable biochemical differences between normal and cancer cells. Already a second metabolic deficiency has been uncovered. It was realized that the preparations of asparaginase could be of benefit clinically despite negative tests in the laboratory. It has been found that, in at least some instances, an additional anti-cancer substance (another normal enzyme, glutaminase) is present in the original, relatively crude, preparations. Developments arising from this exciting new approach are eagerly awaited.

On the other hand, there is every reason to believe that more effective use can be made of presently available anti-cancer drugs which act on normal cells as well as on malignant. Methods for increasing the affinity of these drugs for cancer cells and thus improving the 'therapeutic ratio' have been pursued for decades. They include exploiting quantitative, rather than qualitative, differences such as increased amounts of non-specific enzymes and differences in the acidity and alkalinity of the tissues. Unfortunately, despite many refinements, the anti-mitotic cytotoxic drugs, e.g. alkylating agents, anti-metabolites and anti-biotics, are all sufficiently toxic to normal cells to limit seriously the doses that can be safely administered. Nevertheless, in general, the higher the dose that can be tolerated, the greater the anti-tumour effect. The aim is to cause as much damage as

197

possible to malignant tissue, with the ultimate goal of completely eradicating every tumour-cell in the body. The associated clinical problems are formidable. It is just not possible to go on giving large doses of cytotoxic drugs because of the cumulative toxic effects. Attempts to overcome the obvious limitations have been made by combining various drugs, and in the timing, and spacing, of treatment. The different classes of cytotoxic drugs have different biochemical actions and therefore differing therapeutic and toxic effects. Thus, a number may be combined in an effort to increase the anti-tumour activity without a parallel increase in toxicity. Such combinations are often synergistic rather than additive. The most successful of the régimes are the use of three, four or five drugs in combination in the treatment of acute lymphoblastic leukaemia, Hodgkin's disease and certain testicular tumours. In major part these régimes owe their success to an exceptionally high standard of general care and meticulous supportive therapy, including repeated platelet transfusions and protection against infection; the latter often amounting to isolation of the patient in special rooms. It is evident, however, that even using combinations of present-day drugs in the full doses in the vast majority of tumours, a sufficiently high percentage of malignant cells cannot be killed even to approach the possibility of achieving a complete cure (see p. 165). The exceptions are choriocarcinoma, Burkitt's tumour and certain tumours of young children such as neuroblastoma and Wilms' tumour.

Anti-cancer drugs act, as a general rule, only upon *dividing* cells, thus any cell which does not attempt to enter division while the drug is present is virtually unaffected. It is therefore important to understand precisely the behaviour of tumour cells. Unfortunately, even today, accurate methods for analysing the characteristics of tumour growth are not available. The rate at which the cells divide can be assessed but it is still not possible to measure wastage due to cell death. The relationship between the frequency of division of tumour cells and normal cells is of extreme importance when drugs are used which are capable of inhibiting mitosis in both types of cell. If vital normal cells divide more frequently than tumour cells then, following a course of cytotoxic drugs, the normal cells will be expected to recover rapidly. Correct spacing of courses of treatment would be expected to reduce the number of malignant cells progressively

198

whilst, if the difference between the doubling rates of normal and malignant was sufficiently marked, the intervals between courses could be long enough to permit the full recovery of the normal body cells. Thus, in *theory*, subsequent courses would not have to be curtailed at all because of cumulative toxic effects on normal body cells. This is the principle underlying the administration of repeated courses of drugs, currently common practice in the treatment of acute lymphoblastic leukaemia, choriocarcinoma and Hodgkin's disease. Following the achievement of a remission of the disease, further courses of drugs are given while the patient is clinically well, and apparently free from disease. Already, in acute lymphoblastic leukaemia in children, remissions of three or four years or more are not uncommon, and it is hoped that with the use of asparaginase even longer remissions will be achieved. If remissions of five years can be obtained with some regularity then there may be a distinct possibility that a proportion of the children may actually be cured. The presently available figures suggest that those who live five years will have a 1 in 2 chance of living ten years, a truly exciting prospect.

In contradistinction to the common situation in which the tumour cells divide less frequently than vital normal cells, some malignant cells may divide more rapidly. In which case, clearly, the tumour would be expected to reassert itself before the normal cells could recover sufficiently from a course of treatment to permit a further course to be given. As the mitotic poisons and the anti-metabolites only affect cells actually in the process of division, a possible therapeutic approach would be to expose the malignant cells to such a drug for a sufficient period of time to affect a high proportion adversely but short enough to spare the majority of normal cells. Clearly the longer the duration of treatment the better; to be most effective it should be given for a period of at least as long as the generation time of the tumour cell. Every tumour cell would then theoretically enter mitosis and be exposed to the cytotoxic effects of the drug.

A further refinement lies in the possibility of giving a drug to arrest both normal and malignant cells at a particular phase of the cell cycle. Division may then be re-initiated by the administration of the appropriate antidote. It is envisaged that if, subsequently, both normal and malignant cells divide in phase, and the cycle times differ sufficiently, it should be possible to

199

select a time when a course of treatment will effect the majority of malignant cells while sparing the normal cells. Obviously there is a most urgent need for detailed information about the life cycles of both malignant and normal cells of various kinds. Until such knowledge provides a logical basis for therapy, it cannot be expected that cytotoxic drugs will realise their full potential.

IMMUNOTHERAPY

The most striking results in the chemotherapy of malignant diseases are obtained in those tumours in which spontaneous regressions are not uncommon. For example: choriocarcinoma, Burkitt's lymphoma, and retinoblastoma. Choriocarcinoma is a homograft, the tumour cells being derived from the cells of the foetus, and, as such, almost certainly it is more easily influenced than, e.g. tumours which arise in the mother's own tissues.

It has been shown in acute leukaemia and Burkitt's lymphoma that those patients surviving longest are by no means those receiving the largest doses of chemotherapeutic agents. Both Burkitt's lymphoma and acute leukaemia may improve temporarily after the administration of human blood serum; in the former, serum from patients who have recovered from the disease may produce striking improvement. Such observations have led directly to the present interest in the possibility that immunological principles may be of relevance in the treatment of cancer. Possibly in these instances treatment merely assists a strong immunological response of the host to the foreign tumour tissue. Immunological mechanisms are clearly unable to destroy large masses of cells but it is quite possible that small numbers, such as remain after successive courses of chemotherapy, or radiotherapy, could be eliminated in this way.

There is a real hope that some forms of cancer (especially any induced by viruses) may eventually be treated, or prevented, by immunological means. Vaccines may prevent actual infection by an oncogenic virus or the later development of overt malignancy. It has been shown experimentally in animals that the suppression of the immune mechanism favours the development of malignant disease and in man there is concern that the administration of immuno-suppressive agents such as are used after kidney transplantation may in certain circumstances encourage the development of cancer in a small proportion of patients. (See Baldwin, p. 108.) The corollary that increasing the immune response is of benefit in restricting cancer growth is presently under test.

The immunological defence mechanism of the patient is likely to be of paramount long-term importance in the control of cancer. The stimulation of patients' defences both in specific, and non-specific, ways may result in a significant reduction in tumour recurrences in patients in whom the bulk of tumour has been eliminated.

R. W. Baldwin has given, in some detail, the ways in which cancer-specific antigens may be sought for in human malignancies and the possibilities for immunotherapy thereafter – both passive and active.

The degree of depression of the immunological reserves in patients with advanced cancer emphasizes the improbability of harnessing the patient's own defence mechanism in the *late* stages of the disease.

It will be appreciated that these are days of high hope in the field of cancer therapy. It seems likely that real advances will come from the study of the more susceptible malignant diseases such as choriocarcinoma, Burkitt's lymphoma and acute lympho-blastic leukaemia. It is of the utmost importance and urgency that these relatively rare diseases should be concentrated in the few centres equipped to provide up-to-date treatment and also in the best position to evaluate further advances as they appear.

THE VALUE OF REGULAR MEDICAL EXAMINATION

Early detection by regular examination has proved itself for selected diseases such as diabetes and pulmonary tuberculosis. It cannot be doubted that in malignant disease also early detection is of vital importance. The belief that regular examinations necessarily cause fear and anxiety has been refuted. In practice such programmes have led to greater co-operation and to a much more realistic outlook over the whole range of medical complaints. In general, from the standpoint of diagnosis and effective treatment, cancer cases may be divided into three categories.

201

The first category includes those cases amenable to early detection and cure, for example breast, cervix, Hodgkin's disease and possibly lung and bladder.

The second includes those cancers which presently often defy detection at a sufficiently early stage to allow the possibility of cure, for example pancreas, stomach and kidney. It is in this group that as new methods of detection are developed the outlook will be expected to change radically.

The third, and luckily much smaller, group comprises those cancers which when first detected are always distributed throughout the body. These are the leukaemias and allied diseases. Nevertheless, if methods were available to detect the earliest cancerous changes almost certainly we would find that the disease process here also arose in a single cell. However in these particular malignancies the position is complicated because many of the cells from which the cancers arise are mobile or invasive in their normal, pre-malignant states. Thus, an abnormal, self-perpetuating series of cells, though originating from one cell in the first instance, would in a matter of hours or days be expected to disseminate itself widely through blood stream and lymphatic channels as a natural consequence of its pre-malignant properties. Nevertheless, even when little can be done to cure, as a rule the earlier disease can be detected the more easily can it be palliated.

There is much to be said for the establishment of early detection clinics open to everyone. Such clinics would have facilities to carry out a complete physical examination, and investigations such as blood counts, X-ray of the chest and the detection of cancer cells shed from certain internal malignancies in particular from the cervix, lung, kidney, bladder, mouth and larynx (exfoliative cytology). Possibly also more specialized techniques, such as mammography and thermography, will be used routinely for the detection of breast cancer. Particularly in cases of cancers requiring more time-consuming, complex and expensive techniques for their detection, it becomes more and more desirable that groups at special risk be defined.

It is well established in laboratory animals that certain states of hormonal imbalance predispose to a wide variety of cancers; this is likely to be so for some cancers of man also. There is presently a major prospective hormonal survey in this country designed to pick out women with the greatest risk of developing cancer of the breast in later years (see Bulbrook, p. 189). Other groups known to be at special risk include those with pernicious anaemia, who have a much greater incidence of cancer of the stomach and certain patients with ulcerative colitis which predisposes to carcinoma of the colon.

The detection of early malignant change, or precancerous states, only helps the patient if the condition can be cured, arrested, or reversed. A good example is carcinoma of the cervix which may be completely removed surgically. On the other hand, in the case of leukoplakia, a widespread pre-malignant condition of the mucous membranes of the mouth, extensive excision is not possible. Sometimes an underlying causative disease for this, such as syphilis, can be treated and the leukoplakia halted but often the changes constitute an almost inescapable hazard of a particular habit, such as the chewing of betel nut, and to attempt to reverse the process would mean an almost unacceptable change in the way of life. Nevertheless, even when little can be done to prevent the development of malignancy the earlier it can be detected the more easily it can be treated.

If the survival rates of patients whose cancers were diagnosed and treated while asymptomatic are compared with those treated after symptoms developed, the value of regular medical examinations can be well justified. In breast cancer an improvement of 25 per cent in the five-year survival figures is achieved. In the cancers of colon and rectum, 35 per cent; uterine cervical cancer, 30 per cent; and in cancers of the body of the uterus, 20 per cent. It has been calculated that, in the USA alone, the general application of the diagnostic and therapeutic skills now available would result in the saving of 80,000 lives each year. It has been estimated that a million persons die each year from cancers which could have been detected whilst still at a curable stage had they been seen, and competently investigated. It is the experience of established cancer-prevention clinics that one treatable cancer is discovered for every 100–150 examinations. It is often argued that the cost of such schemes in time and money would prohibit their application, but it has been shown many times that the results make good economic sense. In this country it is accepted that in specialized sites, particularly the breast and cervix, the results justify the efforts. Although, at the present time, the results of the screening of other sites are not so reward-

203

ing, the position will change and the principle of regular medical examinations and investigation whilst still in good health will gain ground.

The training of doctors and other medical personnel and the expansion of health facilities in general is not, however, keeping pace with the population explosion. Further, an ever greater proportion of the human race is living to an age when cancer is most prevalent. The proportion of doctors' time and skill devoted of necessity to the treatment of cancer increases as the disease spreads and progresses. Regular routine examination would relieve the community of much of the greater burden of caring for far advanced cancer and, as such, would make a significant contribution to the economy. In addition, well designed regular screening programmes would allow epidemiological studies and thus, the definition of high-risk groups; increase our knowledge of the natural history of malignant disease and permit the evaluation of the results of treatment. Important by-products of cancer detection examinations is the discovery of conditions, other than cancer, requiring treatment. Hypertension and other cardiovascular diseases, diabetes, tuberculosis, thyroid disorders and anaemias are found in up to one-third of all patients examined. The outlook in many of these cases can also be improved by early treatment. The mere recording of the 'normal' for any particular patient can be of great value when interpreting changes arising in any future illness. Better health results in greater enjoyment of life, increased productivity and a reduction in demand on the general medical services.

The proportion of our national wealth utilized for the maintenance of health is low in comparison to that of a number of other countries. There is however an increasing awareness that the health of the population is the most important asset of a country. The ill, the disabled and the unfit achieve less than the healthy in mind and body. Slowly, but surely, this view must be fostered so that we as a country will not fall into the slough of mediocrity. The ultimate control of cancer must be based on prevention, but until that day, certain but distant, the early detection by periodic examinations and screening programmes must be encouraged.

THE CONTROL OF CANCER OF THE BREAST

Much can be done towards controlling this common cancer. It is disquieting that a recent survey has shown that as many as 10 per cent of new cases are still, by modern standards, not being adequately treated when they first present, even allowing for the fact that there is some room for debate as to what constitutes the best forms of treatment. A number of controlled trials are in progress designed to reduce many of the uncertainties but there is need for more co-operation between centres so that decisive answers can be obtained without avoidable delay. In practice, patients often do very much better than might be expected; much might be learned from a study of this responsive group.

Work is also under way to attempt to detect a metabolic abnormality which antedates, and may possibly predispose, to the development of breast cancer (see Bulbrook, p. 189). If it proves possible to pick out a group of women with a special risk an enormous new field would open up. Perhaps such a predisposition could not be corrected but at least the group could be kept under close observation. There remains the very real possibility of eventually uncovering important environmental factors. Japanese women have a much lower incidence of breast cancer than European, or American, women; yet following emigration to the United States of America and the adoption of western dietary and other habits the next generation become more prone to the disease. This observation, if explained, might suggest means by which the incidence could be reduced.

All women should be taught to examine their breasts regularly and to seek advice if an irregularity is noticed. Early diagnosis is vital and many hospitals now have special clinics known as Well Women Clinics devoted to the detection of cancer of the breast and cancer of the uterine cervix at the earliest stage possible with modern techniques.

Recent years have seen the development of new and more precise ways of detecting cancers of the breast. These include special X-ray techniques (mammography) and measurement of thermal activity (thermography). It is clear however that even using modern techniques screening examinations would have to be carried out more than once a year. The importance of defining those at special risk thus becomes an urgent necessity.

THE CONTROL OF CANCER OF THE CERVIX

This serious and common cancer develops in women in the prime of life. Even with the latest methods of radiotherapy and the most radical surgery there has only been a marginal increase in survival rates over the past decade. Thus, the emphasis has passed to early diagnosis. It is a fact that where cervical cytological screening has been organized on a community basis, the incidence of invasive cervical cancer has fallen steadily and there is evidence that the death rate is also falling. Early cases can be detected by these means long before the development of signs or symptoms sufficient to take the patient to her doctor. The cervical smear test itself is quick, simple and quite painless; the actual reading of the smear however is time consuming and highly skilled. There is great need for the development of an automated method. The cervix is a site where such techniques can be most rewarding because the cancer cells are easily accessible. In the very early stages the lymph nodes are never involved, so the patients are curable.

Regional centres are being set up to offer these services to the public. It is evident that the concentration of cases so achieved will, quite apart from the benefit of early diagnosis, lead to the development of more effective forms of treatment. Cancer of the cervix is commoner in the lower social classes. The incidence of the cancer in wives of professional men is only one-fifth that for married women as a whole – a difference attributable to increased standards of living, personal cleanliness and the higher incidence of circumcision of the husbands. The highest yield of cases diagnosed comes from female venereal disease clinics. The organization of cervical smear screening services has been the subject of a study by a special subcommittee of the British Medical Association in 1965. The cost to the community of diagnosing each case is estimated to be between £100 and £150 if all women at risk are examined at five-yearly intervals. The general problems are similar to those outlined for diagnostic or early detection clinics.

The initial response to properly presented publicity may be as

206

high as 50–60 per cent. Again the more educated classes, those at lowest risk, respond best. Forty per cent of the population are insensitive to publicity or persuasion, untouched by advertising and personally-directed literature. Again, ignorance, apathy, fear and a general lack of awareness need to be faced and overcome. There is fear that the test may induce sterility or detect promiscuity, quite apart from the fear of the consequences should an abnormality be detected. The high-risk, lower-class group are the most difficult to reach. They may only respond to personal appeal and to visits from informed individuals equipped to carry out the test in the home. In any event it is essential that if the women have plucked up courage to seek a test they should never be sent away to await appointment. It is well known that they may never return!

Clearly, much must be done before the public is able to benefit from the means of control of carcinoma of the cervix presently available.

THE CONTROL OF CANCER OF THE LUNG

The evidence implicating cigarette smoking as a cause of cancer of the lung is very strong. The Report of the Royal College of Physicians of England (1962) and The Report by the Advisory Committee to the Surgeon General of the United States Public Health Service (1964) are most authoritative and comprehensive reviews on smoking and health. It is not suggested that cigarette smoking is the *only* cause of lung cancer, but it is difficult to avoid the conclusion that it is the major cause and that if the smoking habit could be abolished the lung cancer death rate would be a small fraction of what it is now. Abolition of the habit would also lead to a substantial reduction in bronchitis, duodenal ulceration and heart disease.

A high proportion of smokers find giving up smoking an impractical proposition. For a variety of reasons they find themselves quite unable to do so. Until more is known of the psychology of addiction to allow a realistic approach, it is unlikely they will be persuaded to do so. The young should be actively discouraged from taking up the habit. Advertising must be strictly controlled, for despite recent improvements it is still presented as socially desirable and a sign of maturity. For those already addicted, efforts should be directed towards reducing the total amount smoked, avoiding inhalation and throwing away a long butt. Cigarette smokers should be acquainted with the considerably reduced risks associated with cigar, or pipe, smoking. Not the least among the bars to concerted action is the enormous revenue obtained from tobacco and the size of the labour force involved. The social factors involved here are considered by Mr Wakefield in the next chapter.

The mortality from cancer of the lung is higher in urban than rural areas. It is argued that this is the result of air pollution and that cleaner air would achieve a substantial reduction in the mortality figures. There is no evidence, so far, to substantiate this view : features of town life other than the carcinogenicity of the air could well be responsible. Nevertheless this is no reason for not taking all practical steps to reduce air pollution to a minimum.

CANCER OF THE DIGESTIVE TRACT

Perhaps one of the most difficult, and least well treated, forms of malignant disease is carcinoma of the hypopharynx and upper oesophagus. So often, by the time the patient reaches the surgeon, the growth is no longer confined to the food passages but has spread to the adjacent tissues and lymph nodes of the neck and mediastinum. It is well known that long-term deficiency of iron predisposes to the development of cancer in this region. Changes in the membranes of the pharynx are usually among the first effects of iron deficiency and occur before the characteristic anaemia. Women are commonly deficient in iron due to the demands of menstruation, pregnancy and lactation and this deficit is not easily met by the modern diet. Nowadays it is modern practice to prescribe iron during pregnancy, and in Sweden iron is added to the flour. Iron deficiency also figures amongst the known predisposing causes of other cancers of the oral cavity including the tongue. Not unusually other deficiencies co-exist, e.g. of vitamins A and B and of protein. Protein deficiency, as will be mentioned later, is also a predisposing factor in cancer of the liver. Other local factors, often avoidable or reversible, include the many forms of chronic inflammation whether of infective, chemical or physical origin. The constant mechanical

208

injury of the tongue from a broken tooth and syphilitic inflammation are often quoted examples. In the East the most important cause of cancer of the mouth is the habit of chewing mixtures of tobacco, lime and betel nuts (Bhang, Khaini). Ceylon has the unfortunate distinction of having the highest death rate from oral cancer in the world (approximately 16 per 100,000 per year). The betel-nut habit is part of the oriental way of life. It is a source of solace and pleasure cheap enough to be widely enjoyed by the underprivileged. Obviously it will be very difficult to persuade these to give up one of their few pleasures and there is every hope that the habit will die as standards of living improve and the spitting associated with the practice becomes less socially acceptable.

Cancer of the stomach is particularly interesting because it is one of the few cancers actually becoming less common in the civilized world. It is thought that highly spiced foods and poor oral hygiene are predisposing factors. Vitamin B12 deficiency in particular pernicious anaemia, which is the result of failure of absorption of the vitamin due to atrophy of the lining of the stomach, is associated with a greatly increased risk of developing stomach cancer. It is this group which would be the most deserving and rewarding for inclusion in any experimental scheme aimed especially at the early detection of carcinoma of the stomach.

Primary cancer of the liver is common in the underdeveloped countries, particularly in the East and in Africa. It is rare in Britain. Amongst many predisposing causes as mentioned earlier are protein and vitamin deficiencies, overloading with iron and poisoning with aflatoxin (see Baldwin and Matthias, p. 117). There is also an association between the development of liver cancer and infestation with liver flukes which are prevalent in the Far East and Eastern Europe. No effective treatment exists for the established infestation, and control by interfering with its life cycle is a major problem of education and economy. The sterilization of faeces and the cooking of all fish, the obvious points of attack on the parasite's life cycle, cannot be enforced, in part because human faeces are used traditionally in cultivation and because of the scarcity of fuel which accounts for peculiarities of culinary habit.

There are a number of well recognized predisposing causes

of cancer of the large bowel (colon). Particularly at risk are patients with chronic inflammatory changes involving the whole of the colon (ulcerative colitis). The risk does not assume major proportions until the colitis has been established for ten years or more. Thereafter it increases with time. As there is considerable difficulty in recognizing that a malignant change has occurred it is now generally agreed that in this high risk group prophylactic removal of the colon is indicated. Familial polyposis is an example of a genetic predisposition to, or predetermination of, cancer. The tendency to develop large numbers of polyps of the colon and rectum is a dominant characteristic which carries with it the virtually inescapable chance of malignant change in the course of time. Prophylactic colectomy is indicated. It is also imperative that the relatives of the patient should be examined because of the nature of the inheritance of the tendency.

THE CONTROL OF CANCER OF THE BLADDER

The risk of bladder cancer in some workers in the chemical, rubber and cable industries has already been discussed but there is still need for constant vigilance since it is quite conceivable that not all the chemical substances in man's environment which are capable of causing bladder cancer have been discovered.

Bladder cancer is one of the commonest forms of cancer in Egypt. The geographic distribution is the same as bilharzia infestation of the bladder and there is a statistically significant association between the two conditions. The eradication of bilharzia is desirable on other counts also, but, unfortunately, it is difficult to achieve. Basically it comes down to effective means of interrupting the life cycle of the parasite such as could be accomplished by the proper disposal of excreta, and the avoidance of contaminated water.

This is yet another example of failure not because of lack of knowledge but because of the impracticability of its application. If the knowledge we already have were to be applied *now* to the control of cancer there would soon be a dramatic fall in the annual number of deaths from the disease. Failure to apply this knowledge cannot be attributed primarily to the doctors and scientists but to society, and Mr Wakefield will discuss this problem in the next chapter.

CHAPTER XI

THE SOCIAL CONTEXT OF CANCER

JOHN WAKEFIELD

How people feel about cancer and how they behave when they see themselves threatened by the disease cannot be discussed simply in terms of here and now. Present attitudes to the disease have their roots in the distant past, some of it surprisingly well charted. From a remarkably well-preserved fossilized tail-bone of a dinosaur in the British Museum, we know that cancer affected forms of life on earth almost 80 million years before any man-like creatures appeared. So, over the whole of Man's brief period of evolution, he has been subject to a fatal disease, only later given the name 'cancer', to which he might fall prey if he survived all the dangerous infections, major accidents and the assaults of his own kind. A thigh-bone of Java Man, *Pithecanthropus erectus*, found in 1891, bears evidence of what was almost certainly some form of bone tumour. These remains are about 400,000 years old.

There is evidence, too, from the earliest historical records. The Ebers papyrus from Egypt, written over 3,000 years ago, records prescriptions for the treatment of ulcers and skin sores, some of them almost certainly cancers of the skin. And the following description, though its like could be found even today in case histories in any hospital in any country in the world, was written by the Greek historian and traveller, Herodotus, about the year 430 B.C.

> 'Atossa had a growth in her breast which was ulcerated and spreading. While the lump had been small, she had been too modest to show it to anyone. Now, since it had become worse, she consulted Democedes.'

The unwise woman, Atossa, was the queen of Darius, King of the Persians. Democedes was a captured Greek physician who had risen to a position of wealth and influence at the Persian court after successfully treating Darius for a broken leg when other doctors had failed. The facts of this story are still all too familiar : a woman finding a lump which she knows to be abnormal, putting off action until forced by pain or other unpleasant developments and, in so doing, possibly forfeiting her chances of cure.

There was precious little to offset the black side of the cancer story until the recent years. The discovery of X-rays and radium only came towards the end of the nineteenth century, and the *controlled* used of ionizing radiations in treating cancer did not become established practice on any scale until the 1930s. It was not until after the Second World War – and largely as a result of research in the radar field – that megavoltage X-ray machines were developed which could tackle deep-seated cancers. The surgical treatment of cancer also owed much to the general advances in surgical techniques enforced by two world wars. Many operations that are now performed routinely for cancer would not have been possible before the advent of blood transfusions, antibiotics and the newer anaesthetic techniques. Only in recent years have doctors been in a position to cope satisfactorily with some common forms of cancer; but lamentably few people are as yet aware of the extent of successes in dealing with this group of diseases. Thus, the whole of the more hopeful side of the history of malignant disease has been compressed into the past fifty years or less. With such a short period for the first flickerings of hope to offset many centuries of bitter experience of this hitherto uncontrollable disease, it is not surprising that modern investigators have described the widespread fear of cancer as 'the reflection of a kind of cultural fear – a herd instinct rooted in prejudice and ignorance', and have drawn attention to the 'magical, moral and retributive elements' in our attitudes to cancer. This, then, is the background against which we have to consider why people think as they do, and act as they do, when confronted with the threat, real or imaginary, of cancer.

It is sometimes argued that fear is a perfectly normal reaction to danger and a necessary part of our defensive mechanisms, that fear is what makes us go to the doctor, when illness threatens. This is true, but, when fear exceeds a certain tolerable level for the individual or when he sees no quick way out of his predicament, he either backs off or pretends the danger isn't there. He retreats from the reality of the unbearable situation and takes refuge in convincing 'reasons' for doing nothing, or dismisses the problem totally, if only temporarily, from his mind. Often he will persist in, even step up, the activity which he knows to be harmful. The ultimate effect of extremes of fear is a total inability to act at all. It is the negative responses to fear that occur in so many people where cancer is concerned and lead to delay in seeking treatment. In the end, the onset of pain or increasingly unpleasant symptoms may alter the sufferer's priorities. The urgent need to get relief will override the awful prospect of having his worst fears confirmed. Often those fears are proved to be pointless when the symptoms are found to be caused by something other than cancer. But when cancer *is* diagnosed, the delay may already have been fatal. For those who still think that nothing useful can be done for them if they develop a cancer, Matthew Arnold's lines must seem peculiarly and disturbingly apt :

> Nor bring to watch me cease to live
> Some Doctor, full of phrase and fame
> To shake his sapient head and give
> The ill he can not cure – a name

There is often something more primitive at work than plain inability to face up to the situation. Names have always had a magical force; they still have in primitive societies, and some of this magic remains in our own minds. People have some vague preconceived notion of the sort of person a baby christened Arnold, Jasper or John will turn out to be, and they choose accordingly. Cancer has for long been synonymous with horror and death, and since in magical beliefs the name and thing are one, it is scarcely surprising that so many people will by all possible means avoid having a name given to their fears.

This is all very disturbing and difficult to accept for people whose work is founded on the assumption that reason can triumph over ignorance and old superstitions. But unless their existence is recognized, we are led to an over-simplified view of the problems – and one that will almost certainly give rise to solutions with a built-in failure factor. We may plan and hope for the eventual triumph of reason as it is gradually borne in

213

on a frightened public that medical science really can offer something to outweigh the age-old and once well-founded fears. But it does not help to ignore the fact that more is involved than simple lack of information. At the moment, the scales often seem too heavily weighted against the man who finds a disquieting symptom : he sees no great advantage in seeing a doctor if he thinks nothing can really be done for him. It is one of the crucial points of current attitudes to cancer that people are not convinced they will be better off if they seek treatment quickly when worrying symptoms arise. And until they are convinced, they will feel no sense of urgency in seeing a doctor.

Two factors work against the growth of public confidence. One is what happens to the patient with incurable cancer; the other is the generally accepted idea that it is better for the doctor 'not to tell'. Cancer in its later stages is commonly thought of as inevitably a painful and distressing condition about which the doctor seems to be doing very little. Often, too, treatment is dismissed as inept or useless. But its seeming failures are not always due to inherent flaws in the methods used. They look like failures because ordinary people have never been made aware of the difference between treatment which is designed to cure and that which has no other purpose from the outset than to prolong life or to make the patient more comfortable. Palliative treatment of this kind is mistaken for curative treatment, and when it does not eradicate the disease – which the doctors had never expected it to do – it is regarded as a failure. Sympathetic handling of the patient and adequate information for the relatives, skilled help with the often onerous business of nursing at home, and the proper relief of pain for those who cannot be cured, are therefore vital if there is to be any improvement in the present melancholy image of this disease in the public mind. Everyone knows the dismal side of the picture, has heard of depressing mortality rates or, more strikingly, has had a relative or friend die of cancer. But this gloomy knowledge is not offset by any general awareness that thousands of people every year do recover after treatment and go on to lead normal and fruitful lives. Those who do get well either don't talk about it or, more often, have not been told what disease they were treated for.

In a large cancer treatment centre in Manchester, patients treated successfully for early cancers with every hope of cure

214

were afterwards told what they had been treated for. Two-thirds welcomed this frank acknowledgment by their doctors of what they had almost all suspected, and they were glad that the game of make-believe on both sides was over. But others found it disturbing to be told. For a few, the information was intolerable and was erased from conscious memory. At a later interview, they insisted that they had never been told they had had cancer. Unfortunately, even though the majority welcomed this new honesty on the part of their doctors, we cannot draw general conclusions about telling all patients – at least, not in the present climate of opinion about cancer. So long as a third of all patients may be disturbed in greater or lesser degree by being told, the decision in each case must be left to the doctor in charge. This is a delicate part of the relationship between doctor and patient that does not lend itself to generalizations, however well-meaning. There can be no doubt, however, that, so long as the great majority of cured people do not know or, more accurately, have not been told officially, they have got over an attack of cancer, it will be difficult to promote a wider public confidence in the efficacy of present treatments.

It is unfortunate that an unrealistic view of the possibilities of dealing with certain forms of cancer is not confined to the lay public. Not all doctors know what kinds of survival rates are now being achieved. However skilful he may be, the family doctor is unable, from his own experience, to get a broad perspective of the chances of dealing with particular forms of cancer. For, common though we think the disease to be, a doctor with some 2,500 patients on his list will, on average, see no more than eight new cancer patients each year. From such small numbers, he is simply not in a position to see the whole pattern of success and failure in the treatment of the various forms of cancer. He can read and hear lectures on up-to-date methods and about percentage survival rates; but his personal experience of what happens to his own patients is, not surprisingly, what is impressed most sharply on his mind. Often this view will be clouded by the very discouraging results of treating, say, lung or stomach cancers.

To bring this problem into sharper focus, it is useful to consider the results of a study in Manchester in 1967 among final-year medical students, who might reasonably be expected to have up-to-date knowledge of the outlook for early treatable cancer, and among a number of general practioners. The question, put to them without notice and with no opportunity of refreshing their memory or of consulting others, was : 'Of 100 middle-aged people with the following diseases, how many would you expect to be alive and well five years after treatment?' They were asked to ring one of the numbers 0, 25, 50, 75 or 100. Two of the listed diseases were early cancer of the neck of the womb and early seminoma (a form of cancer) of the testis. For cancer of the neck of the womb, about a quarter of the medical students and a third of the general practitioners forecast 50 or fewer survivors. For the testicular tumour, over 60 per cent of the students and over 80 per cent of the general practitioners forecast 50 or fewer survivors. The nearest correct answer in each case would have been 75 survivors. Because of the way the question was framed, we may assume that some who were uncertain guessed at somewhere around the halfway mark (50 survivors), but there were enough who forecast 25 or fewer survivors to indicate a disquieting degree of misinformation among medical men about the likely outcome for these highly manageable forms of early cancer. Attitudes based on such beliefs must inevitably rub off on patients, relatives and the general public, whose existing fears are thereby reinforced. And a doctor with an unjustifiably pessimistic view of the outcome of treatment may sometimes be a source of further delay in getting an apprehensive patient to the place where he can receive specialist treatment.

Nurses, particularly those engaged in public health work, also play an important part in shaping public attitudes to cancer, since people often talk more freely to them than they do to doctors. Are they able to do something to remedy the dismal general view of cancer? Apparently not. A survey of nearly 800 nurses in public health – health visitors, midwives and district nurses – included questions about the effectiveness of treatment for certain highly manageable early cancers. Their answers laid bare an even more depressing view of cancer than that of the general public. This was not what might have been expected of women with a great deal of professional training and specialized knowledge. But the study made it quite clear that their attitudes were moulded much more by personal experiences of cancer in their families or in their immediate circle and, perhaps, by their daily work *after* training, which necessarily restricts their professional contact with the disease almost entirely to visiting and looking after patients with distressing late symptoms or dying of cancer at home. This side of things is not offset by regular contact with the successes of cancer treatment, for those who get well and require no special nursing after leaving hospital do not come under the professional care of public health nurses.

What, then, can be done to alleviate this depressing burden of fear that leads to delay and, in too many cases, to needless death? If it is a matter of people being uninformed or mis-informed, can we not quite simply set the matter right by supplying them with reliable information? No one would argue seriously against putting out more information, but it would be absurd to assume that this is all that is needed to put things right. Ignorance of the true state of affairs *can* be dangerous or lead to unwise action, or inaction; but there is no evidence whatever to suggest that acquiring new knowledge will, on its own, auto-matically change the habits of a lifetime. Yet this naïve view of health education about cancer has been put forward by a number of professional men who ought to know better. When the word 'ignorance' is used in this context, it carries with it a flavour of puritanical disapproval, a suggestion that the lower orders really ought to try harder to rid themselves of their self-imposed handi-caps. Or even worse, it insults by its condescending assumption that 'they' ought to leap at the chance 'we' offer to fill up all those empty spaces in 'their' minds. But people do not have blank spaces into which doctors and health educators can slip desirable information. They have their own system of beliefs about the way diseases arise and how, if at all, they can be dealt with. Some signs and symptoms are regarded as threatening, others as of less immediate importance. The professional may know that some of these beliefs are unscientific and that some are positively harmful, but holding beliefs of this kind is very different from having no beliefs on the subject at all.

There as still some bizarre, and fortunately less commonly-held, beliefs about what may cause cancer: tomato seeds, tight corsets, plastic teacups and aluminium pans are examples. Yet even today, in England about 1 woman in every 5 thinks that cancer is inherited, that it is 'catching' like influenza, caused by

217

an immoral way of life, or by the knocks and bumps that are part of our everyday life. These, at least, were the figures to emerge from the report, published in 1967, of a sample survey of women in Lancashire, and they do not differ greatly from studies that have been done in other places. One of the most striking features of these beliefs is their fatalism and the element of divine retribution that is so often to be found in the folklore of diseases which are little understood and regarded as inevitably fatal. We all like to think of ourselves as rational beings, but there are darker sides to all our minds, where new knowledge is not always strong enough to fight off old terrors and superstitions. Though we may not recognize it in such precise terms, a tendency to fatalism emerges in many of us, especially at times of special stress or when confronted with something we know little about and feel we cannot control. In psychological terms, this could be explained as a way of avoiding responsibility for what follows by resigning ourselves to the situation. But it can also occur in people who do act as best they can in the circumstances, who use their knowledge to take advantage of what medical science can offer. In them, it may be the result of something more powerful and more primitive – a sense that there is some mysterious force at work controlling our destinies. It is not the place here to debate the form this may take, though it is obvious that those who hold religious beliefs will recognize this force in more particular terms. It is enough for the present purpose to understand that fatalism cannot easily be dismissed as the simple concomitant of ignorance.

The extent to which cancer is still regarded as wholly incurable was shown in the Lancashire survey. Older women – who are, of course, so much closer to the problem – take a gloomier view than the young : only 53 per cent of the over-60s, compared with 77 per cent of the under-40s, believe that cancer can sometimes be cured. And those at the lower end of the socio-economic scale take a notably more pessimistic view than those at the upper end. The greatest range of differences is seen when we compare women over 60, married to semi-skilled and unskilled workers, with women under 40, married to men in white-collar and professional jobs. Only 42 per cent of the former believe that cancer can sometimes be cured as against 93 per cent of the latter.

218

All these statements involve comparisons of the differences between what people engaged in health education accept as appropriate concepts and what the man and woman in the street believes. The professionals define health and illness according to up-to-date medical knowledge and, since they must necessarily take a broad view of the problems, their definitions tend to rely on the patterns that emerge from studies of whole populations. Such populations may consist of all the inhabitants of a country, or a region where peculiarities have required investigation, of occupational groups exposed to special risks, or of groups with habits known to have long-term effects on health. But the man in the street takes a much more personal view of health and illness. It is not the broad patterns that interest him : it is how illness will affect him and his family, his ability to earn and his freedom to do those things he is accustomed to doing.

To health professionals, the man in the street behaves in an unreasonable manner if he does not go to a doctor when certain well-publicized signs and symptoms crop up, or if he fails to take advantage of preventive and detection tests made available and advertised by the authorities. Yet going to see a doctor may seem an entirely *un*reasonable act to the otherwise healthy person with a seemingly trivial symptom. Doing something about it may – for some time, at least – take a very low priority behind keeping a job, not taking time off work and reducing earnings, not falling behind on hire purchase or house mortgage payments, or keeping up the standards of his own particular community, which may set a very low value on those who give in easily to complaints that are not obviously incapacitating.

What people regard as important in matters of health differs from one section of the community to another. Most people would regard a sore throat as a fairly minor irritation; to singers it may be disaster. Tennis elbow would not stop a computer programmer from working; it could stop a bricklayer or a miner from earning a living. These are deliberately obvious examples, but similar, if less instantly recognizable, factors are at work in all our decisions (if that isn't too strong a word) on matters of health and disease. A one-man business comes to a halt if the owner falls ill. On a small farm someone has to feed, water and milk the cows, tend the ewes at lambing, and so on. They cannot be left to fend for themselves because the farmer feels out of

219

sorts or because his wife has found a small lump that isn't causing pain or interfering with her capacity for work. This kind of life demands that people carry on as long as they can, and in remote agricultural communities it has bred a stoicism that allows no one to give up work save for some major physical handicap. In this setting, well-meaning advice about seeing the doctor for things that don't interfere with work is not only ineffective, it is fatuous. Where posters, pamphlets and persuasion would fail, finding someone to tend the cattle might succeed. At least it would offer a way out of the problem that looms so large in the farmer's mind that other personal worries are submerged until they progress to something more drastic.

A classic example of the way interests conflict in the individual and in society is in our attitude to the cause of the great plague of modern times – cigarette smoking. It is beyond any reasonable doubt that people who do not want to develop lung cancer, bronchitis, or coronary heart disease can greatly reduce their risk of doing so by not smoking cigarettes. Lack of knowledge isn't a problem – the Government Social Survey's report in 1968 showed that 93 per cent of the population over school age in Britain knew of the link between cigarette smoking and health hazards – yet over 60 per cent of all men still smoke cigarettes. But we cannot ignore the fact that many of those who smoke derive pleasure from doing it, and everyone knows the powerful social pressures that work against anyone trying to give it up. Until something occurs to bolster their resolve, smokers puff on regardless, putting their terrifying knowledge out of mind in favour of the immediate 'advantages' they derive from smoking. This, at least, is one point at which doctors and other health professionals who still smoke are confronted rudely with their own frailty. Although they are members of an élite group with access to all the weighty scientific evidence against cigarettes, they ignore it and behave exactly as the erring individuals whose unreasonable behaviour they lament in other, and often less clear-cut, situations.

The background is very similar when we consider the problems involved in mounting a screening programme to examine outwardly healthy women by means of cervical smears. From the medical point of view, discovering conditions that may go on to become true cancer if left untreated is even more desirable than detecting early cancers. For the first time, doctors have an

220

opportunity of dealing with a *pre*cancerous condition and, they believe, preventing it by comparatively simple methods from progressing to something much more serious. Despite the reservations of those who believe that not all these precancerous conditions go on to become cancer and that not all cancers of the cervix are necessarily preceded by a lengthy non-malignant phase, most doctors who are involved in treating this form of cancer have welcomed the introduction of this simple test as a promising way of cutting down the number of needless deaths.

It might be thought that the general public would be even more eager to welcome a test designed to prevent the onset of cancer. In a general way, this is true. Cervical cytotests are regarded as a good thing, and there has been a great deal of public pressure from influential women's organizations to have the tests made available to women all over the country. But making approving noises is one thing; going to have the test oneself is quite another. Paradoxically, the reason why the cytotest is so attractive to doctors – because it reveals indications of possible future trouble long before there are any outward signs or symptoms – is why some women are even less inclined to volunteer for examination that they are to go to a doctor when symptoms appear. A woman who has no hint of illness, no unexpected bleeding, no discharge, does not feel herself threatened by disease. And she certainly doesn't want the test to show she has cancer or the forerunner of it. To see the value of the cytotest, she has to have been brought up in an environment where thinking ahead and planning for the future, whether in matters of finance or health, is accepted as normal. If she has not – and it is still one of the hard facts of working-class life that getting through today is the main preoccupation – she will find it hard to see the long-term advantages and may be put off by the practical business of making and keeping an appointment at a clinic. In one of our studies, out of 600 women who came of their own accord to have a cytotest at a clinic, 112 failed to turn up for the appointment they were given. Booking arrangements that seem simple and informal to those who devise them may be confusing and unfriendly to the woman they are intended to help. Even more formidable is the alternative of raising the subject with her family doctor, when she thinks she has no real justification (that is, when she doesn't regard herself as 'poorly') for

221

visiting him. This is why it is so important for the family doctor to take the initiative in suggesting the test to working-class women who visit his surgery.

How difficult it is for the medically trained, and those whose work is based on the current concepts of medical science, to envisage all the barriers that others lower down the social scale will find in the way of their accepting what seems such a simple, ordinary test, is seen from some recent studies in the USA. A cytological screening programme was launched in part of Florida. The organizers concentrated their efforts on a high-risk group, women receiving state aid for dependent children, poor and with little education. They arranged a vigorous programme of publicity and went to a lot of trouble to send each woman a simple, friendly letter of invitation. The response was very disappointing. A research team went in to try to discover what had gone wrong. Before they could find out anything worth knowing, they had to trace the network of communication by which information was received, circulated and approved in the community. Uncovering this network – there were unofficial leaders of opinion on matters of health, whose endorsement of suggested actions on health matters was needed if others were to co-operate – showed how the generalized publicity campaign had gone wrong in the first place. Next, the carefully worded letter of invitation was found to have been virtually useless. Because of what the investigators called 'functional illiteracy', many of the women simply acquired no information from it. They could read the words but the letter conveyed no message to them. Letters are things you get from 'the authorities', not ways of passing on important information. Anyone who finds this ludicrous might care to recall the effect on himself of some of the explanatory notes enclosed with his income tax return.

As if these difficulties were not enough, even the explanations of what the cytotest involved, and what it was for, turned out to be inadequate. It told all that was needed from the point of view of those who had devised the programme, but it left untouched a number of questions and fears that were crucial to the women concerned. Perhaps the most important was that this was thought of as a 'cancer test', and it was an overriding fear of cancer that kept many women away. The idea that it was a test to find certain disorders that could be prevented from turning into cancer had not been understood. There were other matters – quite unrelated to cancer – that worried the women : would this test interfere with their sex life? Make them less attractive to their men? Would it cause sterility? Would it reveal past sexual misdemeanours that might get back to other people from whom they had been kept secret? and so on.

This Florida programme is not put forward as an awful example of health education planning; in fact it was a careful and important piece of work in which, fortunately, a good deal of care was devoted to checking its progress so that errors could be detected and put right. How successfully this was done may be seen from the subsequent progress of the scheme : in areas where the revised programme was applied, nearly 75 per cent of these poor and ill-educated women were persuaded to take part in the scheme – a greater proportion than is usually achieved among better off and better educated women. The main importance of this anecdote, however, is to show how easy it is for trained professionals to go astray when they plan their work in the basis of their own needs and their own background. 'Common sense' – a sacred cow to the English – is a poor basis for health planning, for it often means no more than what the planner thinks he knows about the people he is planning for.

As other screening measures, now being developed, are brought to an adequate level of efficiency, the central core of the problem will remain. People who undergo the tests will be confronted with the possibility that they may be suffering either from a forerunner of cancer, or with the even less tolerable alternative that they may have an early cancer. This is not an easy prospect to face, particularly for outwardly healthy folk who have no reason to suspect that they may be harbouring a deadly disease. And though it is true to say that cancerous growths can be treated with much greater hopes of success when they are still very limited in extent, no doctor would care to give an absolute assurance that all such conditions could be cured. It is certainly encouraging to learn that the cure rate for many forms of cancer is so much better than we had believed. (Table 5 shows the great differences in the results of treatment when the disease is treated at a very early stage and when it is advanced.) But the individual does not think of his chances in

TABLE 5

Percentage of survivors at 5 years

Site	Stage 1	Stage 4
Larynx	75	5
Lip	85	15
Mouth	60	5
Testis	75	15
Cervix uteri	70	10
Bladder	50	15
Breast	70/75	10

Differences in 5-year survival rates for cancers of various sites treated at early and late stages of development.

terms of percentages. For him, he will either get better or he will die : the percentage is either 0 or 100. However promising the picture may be when seen in broad outlines, the individual sees no sure salvation in a 70 per cent survival-rate, so he has no absolute relief from his mortal fears. He sees what he is offered as at best a partial assurance. To offset this is an advantage – but not an immediately inspiring one – the certain knowledge that there is nothing to gain and everything to lose by procrastination. This consideration clearly weighs heavily with many informed people when they are confronted with inescapable symptoms. But it is not a powerful motivation with those who, as far as they know, haven't a thing wrong with them. To ask them to undergo tests and examinations is to ask them to expose themselves to fears and uncertainties with no guarantee that they will come to no harm if something untoward is discovered. The more successful cancer treatment becomes, the greater our chances of persuading healthy people to submit to examination, because the benefits of doing so will have become obvious. The change, when it comes, will be similar to the sweeping change in public attitudes to tuberculosis, which came with the sudden introduction of antibiotics that could control the disease.

Despite the difficulties involved in getting adequate numbers of the women most at risk to be tested, it seems that cervical cytotests offer one of the best chances so far of changing attitudes to cancer generally. If, by means of a carefully documented programme, it can be shown conclusively that selective screening will reduce the present number of deaths from cancer of the cervix, people will for the first time be able to see that the prevention of one form of cancer is a practical proposition. And some of this new feeling of hope, this slight erosion of the pervading fatalism, will rub off on our attitude to other forms of the disease. Looking at the problem objectively, it may be that the cost of screening all adult women in the country by cytotests could never be justified, since the annual deaths from cervical cancer are only around 2,500, not all of whom could necessarily be saved. But if mass screening is successful, it will be of inestimable value in changing the present climate of opinion and bringing about a major shift towards a more hopeful view of cancer.

The possibility of preventing cancer of the cervix has, not unnaturally, stirred up much emotion. Tackling a disease that attacks mothers in their prime has a profound appeal – and not only to women. Twenty-five hundred may not be many deaths in an annual mortality of over half a million in England and Wales, but it means that 2,500 individual women are taken from their families and friends, often at an age when they can least be spared. Yet no comparable degree of emotion is aroused by an almost wholly preventable form of cancer that kills over ten times as many people annually. It is scarcely believable that we are prepared to accept a number of needless deaths that is equal every year to the annihilation of every man, woman and child in Ilfracombe, Llangollen, Minehead and Penrith. If it were some mystery virus that wiped out nearly 30,000 people each year, the public clamour for action by medical and governmental authorities would be instant and deafening. But lung cancer victims don't all die in one place, and publication of the annual mortality figures for lung cancer cause no more than a mild shudder in the press. The dire warnings of the Chief Medical Officer pass almost as unnoticed as the hell-fire rantings of Hyde Park orators. Our psychological defence mechanisms come smoothly into action, and we reassure ourselves that this is something that happens to people with weak lungs or that dangerously heavy smoking means five or ten cigarettes a day more than we smoke, even though the increased risk of death is 40 per cent for people who smoke less than ten a day.

Much play is still made of the tired argument that the connection between cigarette smoking and lung cancer (as well as heart disease, bronchitis and emphysema) has not yet been proved beyond doubt : that it is only a matter of statistics – as if the statistical demonstration of cause and effect were no more than a sophisticated form of chicanery. To say that a heavy cigarette smoker has one chance in eight of dying of lung cancer seems to leave fairish odds in favour of escaping this fate. But if the problem is presented in some more immediate form, the odds seem much less attractive. If it were known than on one particular airline, one flight out of every eight ends in a fatal crash, how many of us would choose to travel with them ?

There has over the past few years been a slight decline in the proportion of cigarette smokers in the population, but this improvement shows signs of tailing off. It is not for lack of information that there has been no dramatic change in smoking habits, since we know that almost all the adolescent and adult population is aware of the link between cigarette smoking and health hazards. Cigarette smoking, apart from being pleasurable to many, is part of a complicated network of social behaviour, a giving and taking of gifts, a demonstration of friendship and belonging to the community in which it is an accepted part of the social ritual. Huge pressures operate against the individual who wants to opt out. Some are deliberate, such as massive advertising by the tobacco trade and the chaffing of friends who seek to turn the backslider from his nonconformity. Some are less overt but no less powerful, such as his endless exposure to the evidence that most of his friends smoke and enjoy it – at work, at home and in their leisure pursuits. There is, too, the constant demonstration by performers on television programmes of all kinds that smoking is a perfectly acceptable, even desirable, habit. Yet, for all the difficulties, some way surely has to be found, in any society with pretensions to civilization, of halting this needless slaughter. It is irrational to raise a hue and cry about the comparatively minor forms of cancer, while the major preventable killer goes unchecked.

If this recital of the many barriers to sensible action seems depressing, it is not meant to be. Rather, it is an attempt to look realistically at the problems involved, so as to prepare the way for a well-designed assault. Cancer is a deeply emotive topic, and

226

education of the public about it has suffered, and still suffers, from the uncritical enthusiasms of those who care passionately and want to see something done today – or, at the very latest, tomorrow. No one would wish to see these enthusiasts suppressed, for without them nothing would get done. But their activities need to be directed into the right channels if they are to provide fruitful irrigation of a barren field and not be dissipated in clouds of useless vapour. It is no longer enough to dole out information like soup to the poor and hope the recipients will make proper – and grateful – use of it. We have to know the limitations of our material and what stands in the way of people making use of it. Above all, we have to formulate in advance a clear notion of what we hope to achieve by public education and strive constantly to check that what we are doing is having the effects we had hoped for and – of great importance with so delicate a subject – that it is not having any unforeseen harmful effects. It is, for instance, all too easy, in our anxiety to stress the ravages of lung cancer in heavy cigarette smokers, to raise a new bogy in the public mind to add to those nameless terrors of the disease that we are trying to combat by other means.

In general, the wisest course at present seems to be to press for a general programme of health education concerning those cancers with which doctors can deal effectively if treatment is begun when the disease is still limited in extent. The aim should be to change the current climate of opinion to one in which cancer is regarded as just another of the serious diseases, curable at best, and at worst manageable. There must be no sacrifice of truth, for to be caught out in exaggerated claims, even with the best of intentions, is to invite rejection of everything that is said. Nevertheless, it is still possible and necessary to lay more stress on the more optimistic aspects of cancer treatment that remain largely unknown, to do something to counter the depressing recital of annual mortality figures from cancer and the melancholy gossip that wells up around every death from the disease. How many people, for instance, know that the number of people cured annually of cancer in England and Wales is about 30,000? How widely is it known that the cancers come a long way behind cardiovascular diseases in the number of people each kills annually? These and other facts would at least help to diminish the spectre of cancer as the major killer disease against which

227

no treatment is effective. The aim should be to strive patiently for a state of affairs in which it is the normal and accepted thing (by both patients *and* doctors) to seek medical advice as soon as certain warning signs appear, whatever the eventual diagnosis.

The mass media are a most valuable way of spreading information, but the personal methods of communication (lectures and discussions with small established groups in the community, the advice of medical professionals to those they come into contact with, the conversation of informed friends and relatives) offer greater chances of influencing action directly. They are also subject less to the danger inherent in mass communications— that a predetermined and necessarily compressed message, whether on poster, in pamphlet or film, offers no opportunity of having doubts dispelled or obscurities made clear in the mind of the recipient. Incidentally, studies in Canada suggest that television has to be regarded more as one of the personal media of communication in health matters, perhaps because it brings our medical advisers right into the home.

Of all the personal methods of communication on health matters, the words of the doctor to his patient are probably the most likely to influence people's behaviour. This is not the place to debate whether this is a natural response to someone whose special knowledge and authority is accepted when one is in a particularly vulnerable situation, or whether it is a truly educational process which will have a lasting influence on the patient's future behaviour. It is enough to draw attention to the strength of this influence, whether it be immediate or long-term. Not many doctors regard themselves in so many words as health educators. Yet everything they say and do to their patients, even the way in which they respond to sufferers' approaches, is a form of health education. The only question is whether its effects will be for good or ill. This is one area in which undergraduate medical training is sadly lacking, for health education is too often regarded as a job for somebody else and not an integral part of the relationship between doctor and patient. Training, from the earliest days in medical school, needs to make much of the tremendous contributions that doctors can make in the intimate setting of the surgery, consulting room, clinic or hospital, simply by being more aware of what they are saying, how they are saying it, and by considering the probable effects on their patients.

228

The remarks in the preceding paragraph apply equally to nurses. They are in positions of special knowledge and authority, and people often find it easier to speak to them than to their doctors. Nurses in the public health service, meeting people at home or in the clinics, are particularly well placed to influence others. Some have direct responsibility for health education, but it is in the informal contacts that so much valuable work can be achieved. In cytological screening programmes for cervical cancer, nurses can be extremely effective both in persuading women they know to be at risk to have a cytotest, and in making sure that all women who come for the test know exactly what it is for and why re-examination at regular intervals is so important.

Doctors and nurses also play a crucial role in looking after patients in whom the disease has passed beyond the reach of all present methods of curative treatment. Seeing that they are enabled to enjoy the final period of their lives as actively and with as little pain and indignity as possible means a great deal to the patients and to their relatives. In some cases, help with night nursing can lighten the heavy burden of caring for the chronically sick at home. Generous and humane care at this difficult time has wider implications. It can help to do something to offset the very common view that cancer patients are finally sent home from hospital to die agonizingly with no one, other than frantic relatives, showing any particular interest in what happens, until death puts an end to the dreadful episode. This is part of the depressing public image of cancer, and it needs to be corrected as quickly as possible – not by bland assurances, but by letting everyone see that real efforts are being made to provide adequate care for patients at home and their families. The Marie Curie Memorial Foundation has shown the way in Britain, but a great deal still needs to be done to provide adequate services from official sources. The need is too great to be left to charitable organizations to do what they can to patch up governmental deficiencies.

There is much to be achieved, too, in the rehabilitation of those who have recovered from an attack of cancer, after extensive surgery. When this involves the loss of some part of the body (removal of a breast, for instance) or some change in its normal functioning (a colostomy to provide a new means of

229

voiding the bowels), the psychological trauma may be more difficult to overcome than the physical effects of the operation. Such patients need understanding and practical help in overcoming these assaults on their person. For a woman to lose a breast is to suffer a serious attack on her essential femininity. She needs skilled medical care, of course, and reassurance that she can return to a normal life; but just as much she needs practical advice and assistance in getting a special brassiere so that she is not endlessly conscious of her changed contours. This part of treatment—the provision of prosthetic appliances to make good the unavoidable losses due to surgery—is not always given the attention it deserves. Yet it has a vital part to play in the slow process of changing the public view of cancer and in reducing fears of the mutilating effects of treatment, which are known to be a cause of putting off seeking medical advice among some patients.

The reasons why some people seek treatment promptly and some only after long delay are still not fully understood, though there is no doubt that a morbid fear of the consequences inhibits many. Lack of confidence that treatment really can be of help if cancer should be diagnosed is still widespread, as was shown dramatically by a study in Manchester. In a study of patients with potentially curable forms of cancer, the investigators found that the women who had a strong suspicion they might have cancer tended to delay seeing a doctor longer than those who did not suspect cancer.

This might seem at first sight to provide a strong argument against education of the public about cancer, but in fact it was a reflection of a complete unawareness that prompt treatment can affect the outcome. Little improvement can be expected until more people understand that cancer is not one disease but a family of diseases, some still difficult to diagnose at a sufficiently early stage for treatment to be effective or resistant to present methods of treatment, but others highly responsive if the treatment can be started when the disease is still at an early stage of development. Public education is needed (1) via the mass media to provide reliable information about preventive measures and screening facilities as they become available, about the treatments and after-care available, and about the curability of certain forms of the disease, and (2) via the personal means of communication (talks and discussions to small groups, information and reassurance passed on by word of mouth from doctors, nurses and informed lay people) to stimulate sensible action when disquieting symptoms arise, or to provide the necessary persuasion to cut down on harmful habits such as smoking). Persuasion of this kind is highly important, too, in the case of women at the lower end of the social scale, who are most at risk of contracting cervical cancer. Public health nurses, visiting such women in their homes and taking smears on the spot, have been found to be highly effective in reaching those who might otherwise not respond to appeals to visit a clinic or their family doctor.

The overall aim should be to create by all ethical means a climate of opinion that is informed and vigilant and not dominated by exaggerated fears. Without any loss of truth, stress has to be laid on the more optimistic and little known aspects of cancer that are now lost in the welter of mournful gossip about those whom treatment failed to save and the depressing emphasis on the annual mortality figures for all forms of cancer. It has to be accepted that this will be a long, long process involving years of unremitting effort to offset the many centuries of hopelessness that inform all our thoughts and emotions about cancer. Much of the basic education needed may have to begin in school, before the young have had time to become infected with the prejudices and harmful beliefs of their elders. It is a difficult task with many pit-falls for the hasty enthusiast. But carefully planned public education, based on adequate research and checked constantly to see that it is doing what it was intended to do, actively supported by doctors and nurses, is the only certain way of ensuring that the best possible use will be made in the future of the facilities for prevention, diagnosis and treatment available to us.

In the special and urgent problem of cigarette smoking – a health problem that incurs so many more deaths than those due to lung cancer – the solution is unlikely to lie with education and publicity alone. It may help to ban all advertising and other inducements; but the most urgent single need is for governmental action to impose a differential tax on cigarettes, so that everyone may see that authority means business and those who *must* smoke something may gain some economic advantage from turning to less harmful cigars or pipes. Without such a tax,

231

governmental statements on the hazards of smoking are an open invitation to justified cynicism.

Knowledge alone does not conquer exaggerated fears of cancer, so the primary task has to be to strive to produce an attitude of mind that will enable people to receive and accept reliable information. Only when we are able to talk and think as freely about the cancers as about other serious but manageable diseases can we expect to see the dramatic saving of lives that will come when doctors are given the opportunity of treating their patients at a stage when they know they can do most to help them.

NOTES ON THE CONTRIBUTORS

JOHN G. BENNETTE

Hon. Secretary of the British Association for Cancer Research. Information Officer and Hon. General Secretary of the British Cancer Council.

LASZLO G. LAJTHA

Director of the Paterson Laboratories, Christie Hospital and Holt Radium Institute, Manchester. Hon. Reader in Pathology, Manchester University.

ROBERT J. C. HARRIS

Head, Dept. of Environmental Carcinogenesis, Imperial Cancer Research Fund. Chairman of the Experimental Oncology Commission of the International Union against Cancer, Geneva. Hon. Associate Professor of Applied Biology, Brunel University. Author of *Cancer, The Nature of the Problem*.

ROBERT BALDWIN

Director, British Empire Cancer Campaign Research Laboratories, Nottingham. Chairman of the Executive Committee of the British Cancer Council.

JOHN Q. MATTHIAS

Consultant Physician, Royal Marsden Hospital and St Bartholomew's Hospital. Author of *Practical Therapeutics*.

SIR JOHN BRUCE

Regius Professor of Clinical Surgery, Edinburgh University. Past President, Royal College of Surgeons, Edinburgh. First President, British Cancer Council.

ERIC C. EASSON

Director of Radiotherapy, Christie Hospital and Holt Radium Institute. Chairman of the Commission on Cancer Control of the International Union Against Cancer, Geneva.

THOMAS A. CONNORS

Senior Lecturer in Biochemical Pharmacology, Chester Beatty Research Institute.

RICHARD D. BULBROOK

Head, Dept. of Clinical Chemistry, Imperial Cancer Research Fund.

JOHN WAKEFIELD

Head, Dept. of Social Research in Malignant Disease, Christie Hospital and Holt Radium Institute, Manchester. Chairman, Committee on Public Education of the International Union against Cancer, Geneva.

233

INDEX

234

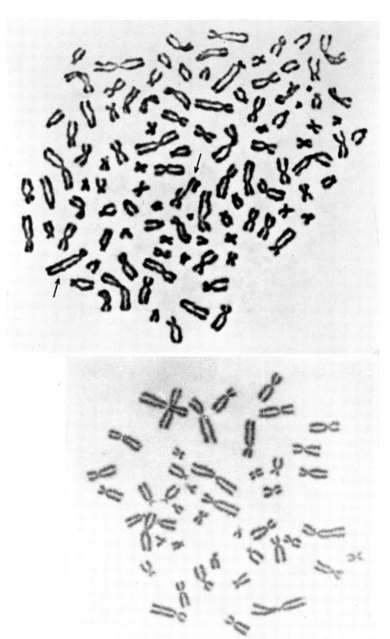

Left, Normal human chromosomes, *right*, chromosomes from a cancer cell. Note the great increase in numbers and also some abnormal or broken chromosomes (arrowed).